Acute Coronary Syndromes

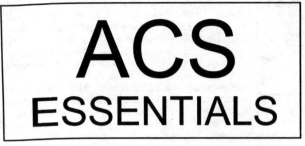

ACS
ESSENTIALS

Robert M. Califf, M.D.

Director, Duke Clinical Research Institute
Professor of Medicine
Donald F. Fortin Professor of Cardiology
Duke University Medical Center
Durham, North Carolina

PHYSICIANS' PRESS

www.physicianspress.com

ROBERT M. CALIFF, M.D.

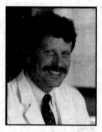

Dr. Califf is Associate Vice Chancellor for Clinical Research, Director of the Duke Clinical Research Institute, Professor of Medicine and Donald F. Fortin Professor of Cardiology in the Division of Cardiology at Duke University Medical Center, Durham, North Carolina, and one of the world's leading authorities on acute coronary syndromes. He is board certified in Internal Medicine and Cardiology and is a Fellow and member of the Board of Trustees of the American College of Cardiology. As Director of the Duke Clinical Research Institute, Dr. Califf has been responsible for coordinating more than 100 randomized clinical trials, including the TAMI trials, the GUSTO trials, and numerous other trials investigating a variety of therapies for acute coronary syndromes, including PURSUIT, ESPRIT, IMPACT I and II, EPIC, ESSENCE, HERO, and ASSENT. Dr. Califf has contributed more than 600 peer-reviewed journal articles and is an editor of the landmark textbook, *Acute Coronary Care*, section editor of *Textbook of Cardiovascular Medicine,* Editor-in-Chief of the *American Heart Journal*, contributing editor for theheart.org, an online information resource for academic and practicing cardiologists, and a member of the Editorial Boards of *Circulation, European Heart Journal, Heart Lung and Circulation, Journal of Cardiovascular Risk, Journal of Invasive Cardiology,* and *Journal of the American College of Cardiology.* Dr. Califf has served on the Cardiorenal Advisory Panel of the U.S. Food and Drug Administration (FDA) and the Pharmaceutical Roundtable of the Institute of Medicine (IOM). He is Director of the coordinating center for the Centers for Education & Research in Therapeutics™ (CERTs), a public-private partnership among the Agency for Healthcare Research and Quality, the FDA, academia, the medical products industry, and consumer groups. Dr. Califf also serves on the American College of Cardiology/American Heart Association Task Force on Practice Guidelines for Unstable Angina and Acute Myocardial Infarction.

Be sure to visit www.physicianspress.com for a complete list of medical titles, along with topical reviews, self-assessment questions, and other clinical information. Additional copies of *ACS Essentials* can be obtained at medical bookstores, or you can contact us directly at:

Physicians' Press / 620 Cherry Avenue / Royal Oak, Michigan, 48073
Tel: (248) 616-3023 / Fax: (248) 616-3003 / www.physicianspress.com

Printed in the United States of America   ISBN: 1–890114–40–5

TABLE OF CONTENTS

OVERVIEW OF ACS

Ch. 1. Overview of ACS **1**
ST-Elevation ACS 3
   Clinical syndrome 3
   Prevalence 4
   Clinical presentation 4
   Classification 4
   Electrocardiogram 4
   Pathophysiology 4
   Management 5
   Prognosis 5
Non-ST-Elevation ACS 5
   Clinical syndromes 5
   Prevalence 5
   Clinical presentation 5
   Classification 6
   Electrocardiogram 6
   Pathophysiology 6
   Management 6
   Prognosis 7

ST-ELEVATION ACS

Ch. 2. Diagnosis and Evaluation **12**
Diagnosis 12
Symptoms 12
   Typical presentation 12
   Atypical presentations 12
   Silent MI 12
Electrocardiogram 13
   ST-segment shifts 13
   Evolution of ECG 13
   Left bundle branch block 13
   Posterior MI 14
   Paced rhythm 15
   Normal ECG 15
Serum Cardiac Markers 15
   Creatine kinase 15
   Cardiac troponins 15
   Myoglobin 15
Ch. 3. Overview of Management **18**
Reperfusion therapy 18
   Fibrinolytic therapy 18
   Percutaneous coronary intervention . . . 26
   PCI vs. fibrinolytic therapy 26
   PTCA vs. stents 27
   Recommendations 28
General measures 29
   Emergency department 29
   Early hospitalization 30

Late hospitalization (> 24 hours) 30
Post-discharge measures 30
Ch. 4. Interventional Management **33**
Primary stenting vs. PTCA 33
Adjunctive pharmacotherapy for PCI 36
   Preprocedural ("Facilitated PCI") 36
   Intraprocedural 36
Procedural technique 37
Deficiencies of PCI 37
Primary PCI for cardiogenic shock 38
Coronary artery bypass grafting 38
Ch. 5. Fibrinolytic Therapy **40**
Overview of fibrinolytic therapy 40
   Primary goal of therapy 40
   Time-dependent benefits 42
   Limitations of fibrinolytic therapy 42
Indications and contraindications 43
Choice of fibrinolytic agents 44
Adjunctive antithrombin therapy 48
Management of lytic complications 48
PCI strategies after fibrinolytic therapy . . 51
   Rescue PCI for failed fibrinolysis 51
   Immediate PCI 51
   Delayed PCI 52
   PCI for recurrent ischemia 53
New reperfusion strategies for acute MI . . 53
   Fibrinolytics plus GP IIb/IIIa inhibitors . . 53
   Fibrinolytics plus enoxaparin 54
   Recommendations 55

NON-ST-ELEVATION ACS

Ch. 6. Diagnosis and Evaluation **58**
Diagnosis 58
   Unstable angina 58
   Non-ST-elevation MI 58
Symptoms 59
Electrocardiogram 59
Serum cardiac markers 61
Other studies 61
Risk stratification 61
Ch. 7. Overview of Management **63**
Emergency department measures 63
Management based on risk category 67
Hospital management 69
Post-discharge measures 69
Ch. 8. Interventional Management **70**
Early invasive vs. early conservative approach
to revascularization 70
Stents vs. PTCA 73

GP IIb/IIIa inhibitors and PCI 73
Coronary artery bypass grafting 74
Recommendations 74

Ch. 9. Adjunctive Medical Therapy 75
Aspirin 75
Clopidogrel 76
GP IIb/IIIa receptor antagonists 79
Low-molecular-weight heparins 85
Direct thrombin inhibitors 91
HMG CoA-reductase inhibitors (statins) . . 92

Ch. 10. Special Patient Populations 94

NON-MEDICAL THERAPIES, MONITORING, RISK STRATIFICATION

Ch. 11. Non-Medical Therapies & Monitoring
Transfer to facility equipped for PCI 97
Primary PCI 97
Immediate PCI (patent vessel) 98
Rescue PCI for failed fibrinolysis 98
Delayed PCI 98
Coronary artery bypass grafting 99
Intra-aortic balloon pump 99
Temporary pacemaker 100
Permanent pacemaker 100
Implantable cardioverter-defibrillator . . . 101
Pulmonary artery catheterization 102
Intra-arterial pressure monitoring 103

Ch. 12. Risk Stratification 103
Stress test 103
Echocardiogram 104
Holter monitor 104
Signal-averaged ECG 104
Electrophysiology study 104
Cardiac catheterization 105

COMPLICATIONS OF ACS

Ch. 13. Arrhythmias and Conduction Disturbances 109
Sinus tachycardia 109
Sinus bradycardia 110
Sinus pause/arrest 111
Atrial flutter 112
Atrial fibrillation 113
Ventricular tachycardia 114
Ventricular fibrillation 115
Accelerated idioventricular rhythm 116
First-degree AV block 117
Second-degree AV block, Mobitz Type I . 118
Second-degree AV block, Mobitz Type II . 119
Third-degree AV block 120
Isolated hemiblock 121
Right bundle branch block 122
Left bundle branch block 123
Bifascicular block 124

Ch. 14. Ischemic, Mechanical, Other Complications 125
Failed fibrinolysis 125
Left ventricular aneurysm 125
Left ventricular pseudoaneurysm 126
Left ventricular dysfunction (acute heart failure) 126
Left ventricular thrombus 127
Mitral regurgitation, ruptured papillary muscle 130
Mitral regurgitation, ischemic papillary muscle 130
Pericarditis, acute 131
Pericarditis, Dressler's syndrome 132
Recurrent ischemia 132
Reinfarction 132
Right ventricular infarction 133
Rupture, cardiac 134
Shock, cardiogenic 135
Ventricular septal defect 136
Major depression 137

ACS PITFALLS

Ch. 15. ACS Pitfalls 138

DRUG SUMMARIES

Ch. 16. Drug Therapy for ACS 147
ACE inhibitors 148
Adenosine 148
Amiodarone 149
Aspirin 150
Atropine 150
Beta-blockers 151
Calcium antagonists 152
Clopidogrel 153
Dobutamine 154
Dopamine 154
Epinephrine 155
Fibrinolytic agents 155
Furosemide 156
Glucose-insulin-potassium 156
GP IIb/IIIa inhibitors 156
Heparin, low-molecular-weight 157
Heparin, unfractionated 158
Ibutilide 159
Lidocaine 159
Magnesium sulfate 160
Morphine sulfate 160
Nitroglycerin 160
Nitroprusside 162
Oxygen 162
Procainamide 162
Statins 163
Warfarin 163

CONTRIBUTORS

Robert M. Califf, MD
Director, Duke Clinical Research Institute
Professor of Medicine
Donald F. Fortin Professor of Cardiology
Duke University Medical Center
Durham, NC

James J. Ferguson, III, MD*
Associate Director, Cardiology Research
St. Luke's Episcopal Hospital and Texas
Heart Institute
Assistant Professor
Baylor College of Medicine
Clinical Assistant Professor
The University of Texas Health Science Center
Houston, TX

Mark S. Freed, MD
Cardiologist
Editor-in-Chief, Physicians' Press
Royal Oak, MI

Valentin Fuster, MD, PhD†
Director, The Zena & Michael A. Wiener
Cardiovascular Institute
Professor of Cardiology
Mount Sinai School of Medicine
New York, NY

Christopher B. Granger, MD
Director, Cardiac Care Unit
Associate Professor of Medicine
Duke University Medical Center
Durham, NC

Cindy L. Grines, MD‡
Director, Cardiac Catheterization Laboratories
William Beaumont Hospital
Royal Oak, MI

Robert A. Harrington, MD
Director, Cardiovascular Clinical Trials
Duke Clinical Research Institute
Professor of Medicine
Duke University Medical Center
Durham, NC

Stephen C. Hammill, MD**
Director, ECG & Electrophysiology Laboratories
Mayo Clinic
Professor of Medicine
Mayo Medical School
Rochester, MN

Alexandra J. Lansky, MD††
Director, Angiographic Core Laboratory
Cardiovascular Research Foundation
Lenox Hill Hospital
New York, NY

Nancy Allen LaPointe, PharmD
Program Director, Duke CERTs (Centers for
Education & Research on Therapeutics™)
Duke Clinical Research Institute
Durham, NC

L. Kristin Newby, MD, MHS
Co-director, Cardiac Care Unit
Associate Professor of Medicine
Duke University Medical Center
Durham, NC

Robert D. Safian, MD*††
Director of Interventional Cardiology
William Beaumont Hospital
Royal Oak, MI

Gregg W. Stone, MD††
Director of Cardiovascular Research & Education
Cardiovascular Research Foundation
Lenox Hill Heart and Vascular Institute
New York, NY

....

*   Chapter 9, Medical Therapy for Non-ST-Elevation ACS, adapted from Ch. 34, Adjunctive Pharmacotherapy, by Ferguson JJ, Freed MS, and Safian RD, in reference (1), below.
†   Mechanisms of fibrinolysis and atherothrombosis, adapted from Ch. 40, Atherosclerosis and Thrombosis, by Peterson M, Dangas G, Fuster V, in reference (1), below.
‡   Portions of sections on lytic complications, non-medical therapies, risk stratification, ischemic/mechanical complications, adapted from Ch. 4, Acute Myocardial Infarction, by Grines CL, in reference (2), below.
**   Portion of section on arrhythmias and conduction disturbances post-ACS, adapted from reference (3), below
††   Portions of sections on percutaneous coronary intervention, adapted from Chapter 5, Acute Coronary Syndromes, by Lansky AJ, Stone GW, in reference (1), below.
1.   *The Manual of Interventional Cardiology*, 3rd ed, Safian, Freed (eds), Physicians' Press, 2002, Royal Oak, MI.
2.   *Essentials of Cardiovascular Medicine*. Freed, Grines (eds), Physicians' Press, Royal Oak, MI.
3.   *The ECG Criteria Book*. O'Keefe, Hammill, Freed, Pogwizd (eds), Physicians' Press, 2002, Royal Oak, MI.

ACKNOWLEDGMENTS

To accomplish the task of presenting the data compiled in this reference, a small, dedicated team of professionals was assembled. This team focused their energy and discipline for many months into typing, revising, designing, illustrating, and formatting the many chapters that make up this text. I wish to acknowledge Rebecca Smith, Monica Crowder-Kaufmann, and Alexis Radulovich for their important contributions. I would also like to thank the many contributors and reviewers who graciously contributed their time and energy amidst busy professional lives, including Sunil V. Rao, MD, Thaddeus R. Tolleson, MD, Christopher K. Dyke, MD, David F. Kong, MD, Eric Valazquez, MD, Darren K. McGuire, MD; Penny Hodgson, Director of Communications, Duke Clinical Research Institute, for researching information, coordinating communication between contributors, and proofreading; Norman C. Lyle, for cover design; and Mark S. Freed, MD, President and Editor-in-Chief of Physicians' Press, for his vision, commitment, and guidance.

Robert M. Califf, M.D.

NOTICE

*We dedicate this volume to the memory
of our Duke colleague, Gary Dunham, RPh,
whose knowledge about the pharmacopoeia
made us all better doctors and was surpassed
only by his caring about the patients
we all shared.*

ABBREVIATIONS

ACC	American College of Cardiology	IV	intravenous
ACE	angiotensin converting enzyme inhibitor	IVCD	intraventricular conduction delay
ACLS	advanced cardiovascular life support	kg	kilogram
		L	liter
ACS	acute coronary syndrome	LAD	left axis deviation
ACT	activated clotting time	LAFB	left anterior fascicular block
ADP	adenosine diphosphate	LBBB	left bundle branch block
AF	atrial fibrillation	LDL	low-density lipoprotein
AHA	American Heart Association	LMWH	low-molecular-weight heparin
AIVR	accelerated idioventricular rhythm	LOS	length of stay
APC	atrial premature contraction	LPFB	left posterior fascicular block
aPTT	activated partial thromboplastin time	LV	left ventricular; left ventricle
		LVEF	left ventricular ejection fraction
ARDS	adult respiratory distress syndrome	LVH	left ventricular hypertrophy
		max	maximum
AV	atrio-ventricular	mcg	microgram
BP	blood pressure	mcL	microliter
BUN	blood urea nitrogen	mg	milligram
CABG	coronary artery bypass grafting	MI	myocardial infarction
CAD	coronary artery disease	min	minute
CCS	Canadian Cardiovascular Society	mL	milliliter
CCU	coronary care unit	MR	mitral regurgitation
CK-MB	creatine kinase-MB isoform	NSAID	nonsteroidal anti-inflammatory drug
CNS	central nervous system		
CO	cardiac output	NCEP	National Cholesterol Education Program
COPD	chronic obstructive pulmonary disease	NPO	nothing by mouth
		NYHA	New York Heart Association
CPK	creatine phosphokinase	O$_2$	oxygen
CPR	cardiopulmonary resuscitation	PA	pulmonary artery
ECG	electrocardiogram	PAI	plasminogen activator inhibitor
Echo	echocardiogram; echocardiography	PaO$_2$	pulmonary artery oxygen saturation
EF	ejection fraction	PAR	plasminogen activator receptor
e.g.	for example	PCI	percutaneous coronary intervention
EP	electrophysiology		
ET	endotracheal	PCWP	pulmonary capillary wedge pressure
g	gram		
GI	gastrointestinal	PE	pulmonary embolism
gm	gram	PET	positron emission tomography
GP	glycoprotein	PO	per os - by mouth; oral
HDL	high-density lipoprotein	PTCA	percutaneous transluminal coronary (balloon) angioplasty
HIT	heparin-induced thrombocytopenia		
		PVR	pulmonary vascular resistance
IABP	intra-aortic balloon pump	q__h	every __ hours
ICD	internal cardioverter-defibrillator	q__d	every __ days
ICH	intracranial hemorrhage	qmonth	once a month
INR	international normalized ratio	qweek	once a week
ISA	intrinsic sympathomimetic activity	QT$_c$	corrected QT interval

RA	right atrium; right atrial	TFPI	tissue factor pathway inhibitor
RAP	right atrial pressure	TLR	target lesion revascularization
RBBB	right bundle branch block	TNK-tPA	TNK-tissue plasminogen
RBC	red blood cell		activator (Tenecteplase)
RCA	right coronary artery	tPA	tissue plasminogen activator
rPA	recombinant plasminogen		(Alteplase)
	activator (Reteplase)	TTP	thrombotic thrombocytopenic
RV	right ventricular		purpura
RVH	right ventricular hypertrophy	TVR	target vessel revascularization
SaO$_2$	systemic arterial oxygen	UFH	unfractionated heparin
	saturation	V/Q	ventilation/perfusion
SK	streptokinase	VF	ventricular fibrillation
SL	sublingual	VPC	ventricular premature contraction
SQ	subcutaneous	VSD	ventricular septal defect
SVG	saphenous vein graft	VT	ventricular tachycardia
SVR	systemic vascular resistance	WPW	Wolff-Parkinson-White
SVT	supraventricular tachycardia	yrs	years
TEE	transesophageal		
	echocardiography		

ACRONYMS

ACUTE	Antithrombotic Combination Using Tirofiban and Enoxaparin
ADMIRAL	Abciximab Before Direct Stenting in Myocardial Infarction Regarding Acute and Longterm Follow-up
APRICOT	Antithrombotic in the Prevention of Reocclusion in Coronary Thrombolysis
ASPECT	Asian Paclitaxel-Eluting Stent Clinical Trial
ASSENT	Assessment of the Safety and Efficacy of a New Thrombolytic
BARI	Bypass Angioplasty Revascularization Investigation
CACHET	Comparison of Abciximab Complications with Hirulog Events Trial
CADILLAC	Controlled Abciximab and Device Investigation to Lower Late Angioplasty Complications
CAMIAT	Canadian Amiodarone Myocardial Infarction Arrhythmia Trial
CAPRIE	Clopidogrel vs. Aspirin in Patients at Risk of Ischemic Events
CAPTURE	Chimeric c7E3 Antiplatelet Therapy in Unstable Refractory Angina
CARS	Coumadin Aspirin Reinfarction Study
CHAMP	Combination Hemotherapy and Mortality Prevention
CLASSICS	Clopidogrel Aspirin Stent International Cooperative Study
CONSENSUS	Cooperative New Scandinavian Enalapril Survival Study
CRUISE	Clinical Revascularization Using Integrilin Simultaneously with Enoxaparin
CURE	Clopidogrel in Unstable Angina to Prevent Recurrent Events
DANAMI	Danish Trial in Acute Myocardial Infarction
DAVIT	Danish Verapamil Infarction Trial
DIGAMI	Diabetes Mellitus Insulin Glucose Infusion in Acute Myocardial Infarction
ELUTES	European Evaluation of Paclitaxel-Eluting Stent
EMIAT	European Myocardial Infarct Amiodarone Trial
EPIC	Evaluation of c7E3 Antiplatelet Therapy in Unstable Refractory Angina
EPILOG	Evaluation in PTCA to Improve Long-Term Outcome with Abciximab GP IIb/IIIa Blockade
EPISTENT	Evaluation of Platelet IIb/IIIa Inhibitor for Stenting
ESPRIT	Enhanced Suppression of Platelet IIb/IIIa Receptor with Integrilin Therapy
ESSENCE	Efficacy and Safety of Subcutaneous Enoxaparin in Non-Q-Wave Coronary Events
FRAXIS	Fraxiparine in Ischemic Syndromes
FRESCO	Florence Randomized Elective Stenting in Acute Coronary Occlusions
FRIC	Fragmin in Unstable Coronary Artery Disease
FRISC	Fragmin During Instability in Coronary Artery Disease
GIPS	Glucose Insulin Potassium Study
GISSI	Gruppo Italiano per lo Studio della Sopravvivenza nell'Infarto Miocardico
GRACE	Global Registry of Acute Coronary Events
GUSTO	Global Use of Strategies to Open Occluded Coronary Arteries
HERO	Hirulog and Early Reperfusion or Occlusion
HOPE	Heart Outcomes Prevention Evaluation
IMPACT-AMI	Integrilin to Manage Platelet Aggregation to Combat Thrombosis
INTERACT	Integrilin and Enoxaparin Randomized Assessment of Acute Coronary Syndromes Treatment
ISAR	Intracoronary Stenting and Antithrombotic Registry
ISIS	International Study of Infarct Survival
MADIT	Multicenter Automatic Defibrillation Implantation Trial

MAGIC	Magnesium in Coronary Disease
MDPIT	Multicentre Dilitiazem Post-Infarction Trial
MIRACL	Myocardial Ischemia Reduction with Aggressive Cholesterol Lowering
MUSTT	Multicenter Unsustained Tachycardia Trial
NICE	National Investigators Collaborating on Enoxaparin
NRMI	National Registry of Myocardial Infarction
OASIS	Organization to Assess Strategies for Ischemic Syndromes
OAT	Open Artery Trial
PACT	Plasminogen Activator Angioplasty Compatibility Trial
PAMI	Primary Angioplasty in Myocardial Infarction
PARADIGM	Platelet Aggregation Receptor Antagonist Dose Investigation and Reperfusion Gain in Myocardial Infarction
PARAGON	Platelet IIb/IIIa Antagonism for the Reduction of Acute Coronary Syndrome Events in a Global Organization Network
PASTA	Primary Angioplasty and Stent Implantation in Acute MI
PCI-CURE	Percutaneous Coronary Intervention — Clopidogrel in Unstable Angina to Prevent Recurrent Events
PRAGUE	Primary Angioplasty in Patients Transferred from General Community Hospitals to Specialized PTCA Units With or Without Emergency Thrombolysis
PRISM-PLUS	Platelet Receptor Inhibition in Ischemic Syndrome Management in Patients Limited by Unstable Signs and Symptoms
PURSUIT	Platelet Glycoprotein IIb/IIIa in Unstable Angina: Receptor Suppression Using Integrilin Therapy
RAPPORT	ReoPro and Primary PTCA Organization and Randomized Trial
RAVEL	Randomized Double-Blind Study with the Sirolimus-Eluting Bx Velocity Balloon Expandable Stent in the Treatment of Patients with de novo Native Coronary Artery Lesions
RESTORE	Randomized Efficacy Study of Tirofiban for Outcomes and Restenosis
RITA	Randomized Intervention Treatment of Angina
SHOCK	Should We Emergently Revascularize Occluded Coronaries for Cardiogenic Shock
SIRIUS	A Multicenter Randomized Double Blind Study of the Sirolimus-Coated Bx Velocity Balloon-Expandable Stent in the Treatment of Patients with de novo Coronary Artery Lesions
SPEED	Strategies for Patency Enhancement in the Emergency Department — Global Use of Strategies to Open Occluded Arteries (GUSTO-IV Pilot)
STAT	Stenting vs. Thrombolysis in Acute Myocardial Infarction Trial
STENT-PAMI	Stent–Primary Angioplasty Myocardial Infarction
STOPAMI	Stent vs. Thrombolysis for Occluded Coronary Stenosis in Patients with Acute Myocardial Infarction
SWIFT	Should We Intervene Following Thrombolysis
SYNERGY	Superior Yield of the New Strategy of Enoxaparin Revascularization and Glycoprotein IIb/IIIa Inhibitors
TACTICS	Treat Angina with Aggrastat (Tirofiban) and Determine Cost of Therapy with an Invasive or Conservative Strategy
TAMI	Thrombolysis and Angioplasty in Myocardial Infarction
TARGET	Do Tirofiban and ReoPro Give Similar Efficacy Trial
TIMI	Thrombolysis In Myocardial Infarction
WARIS	Warfarin-Aspirin Re-Infarction Study
VANQWISH	Veterans Affairs Non-Q-Wave Infarction Strategies In-Hospital

OVERVIEW OF ACS

Chapter 1

Acute Coronary Syndromes

Acute coronary syndromes (ACS) is a term used to encompass the spectrum of clinical disorders caused by acute ischemic heart disease, including unstable angina, non-ST-elevation myocardial infarction, and ST-elevation myocardial infarction, which account for 2 million hospitalizations and 30% of all deaths in the United States each year. Despite major advances in diagnosis and treatment, tens of thousands of lives are lost each year due to delays in diagnosis, failure to implement potent pharmacological and interventional strategies, and inconsistent application of secondary preventive measures. *ACS Essentials* integrates the latest clinical guidelines and trials into a concise, practical, and authoritative guide to the management of acute coronary syndromes.

Initial Classification

Therapeutic decisions are required before patients with ACS can be categorized into unstable angina or acute MI based on serum cardiac markers and serial ECGs. To facilitate early management, patients are classified into ST-elevation ACS or non-ST-elevation ACS based on the presence or absence of ST-elevation ≥ 1 mm in 2 or more contiguous leads on initial ECG. Clinical features and management of ACS are summarized in Table 1.1 and Figure 1.1.

ST-Elevation ACS (Chapters 2-5)

A. **Clinical Syndrome.** ST-elevation ACS has also been labeled "reperfusion-eligible" ACS, since prognosis is improved by early reperfusion with percutaneous coronary intervention (PCI) or fibrinolytic therapy. Patients with left bundle branch block (LBBB) or posterior MI on initial ECG also benefit from reperfusion therapy.

B. Prevalence. 600,000 cases in the United States annually.

C. Clinical Presentation. The most common presentation for ST-elevation MI is chest, neck, or jaw discomfort, which is usually described as pressure, burning, or squeezing in character. Symptoms last ≥ 30 minutes and can occur de novo or in patients with antecedent angina. A precipitating factor is present in 50%. Atypical presentations—weakness, dyspnea, heart failure, dizziness—are more common in women, diabetics, and the elderly. Up to 20% of infarcts go unrecognized by the physician or patient.

D. Classification. Patients with ST-elevation MI are identified by eligibility for reperfusion therapy (Table 5.2, p. 43), infarct location, and associated mechanical, ischemic, or electrical complications (e.g., lytic-eligible patient with anterior MI complicated by ischemic papillary muscle dysfunction with acute mitral regurgitation and heart failure).

E. Electrocardiogram. ST-segment elevation ≥ 1 mm in 2 or more contiguous leads is required for the diagnosis. Unless reperfusion occurs, Q-waves develop in 80%. Patients with LBBB (new or presumably new) or posterior MI caused by left circumflex coronary artery occlusion also benefit from reperfusion therapy. If hyperacute (giant upright) T waves are present, the ECG should be repeated in 15 minutes to identify ST-segment elevation while preparing for reperfusion therapy. For paced rhythms, the pacemaker rate can be reprogrammed below the intrinsic heart rate to detect ST-segment shifts.

F. Pathophysiology (Figures 3.2, 3.3, pp. 23-24). The most common cause of ST-elevation MI is occlusive thrombus that develops at the site of a ruptured or fissured atherosclerotic plaque. Most ruptures develop in moderate (< 70%) stenoses with soft, lipid-rich cores and thin fibrous caps. Without coronary reperfusion, myocardial necrosis begins in the subendocardium and spreads to the epicardium, resulting in transmural infarction, and Q-waves develop on ECG. Even with coronary reperfusion, embolization of atherothrombotic debris can prevent myocardial reperfusion and recovery of left ventricular (LV) function. On coronary angiography, 40% of patients without prior MI or angina have single-vessel disease, 30% have 2-vessel disease, 15% have 3-vessel disease, and 10-15% have no significant obstruction. In contrast, 50% of patients with prior MI or angina have 3-vessel disease and 15% have significant left main obstruction.

G. **Management (Figure 3.1, p. 19).** Acute reperfusion therapy with PCI or fibrinolysis is recommended, depending on the availability of a skilled interventionalist and lytic eligibility. Primary stenting is preferred over balloon angioplasty (PTCA). Adjunctive pharmacotherapy includes aspirin, heparin, beta-blockers, ACE inhibitors, and nitrates; routine use of GP IIb/IIIa inhibitors is reasonable. Recent studies suggest that transfer to a PCI center may be preferred to on-site fibrinolytic therapy, and that "facilitated" PCI with upstream use of low-dose fibrinolytics or GP IIb/IIIa inhibitors may enhance tissue reperfusion; further studies are underway.

H. **Prognosis.** Many patients with acute MI die before seeking medical attention, and another 10% die during hospitalization, for an overall acute mortality rate of 25-30%. The majority of hospital deaths occur within the first 2 days, emphasizing the importance of early intervention. Most deaths that occur in the first year do so within the first 12 weeks, usually in patients with LV dysfunction (EF < 0.40), symptomatic heart failure, complex ventricular arrhythmias, significant residual coronary artery disease, or LV aneurysm. Restoration of coronary blood flow within the first 12 hours of acute MI results in myocardial salvage, preservation of LV function, fewer in-hospital complications (heart failure, pulmonary emboli, arrhythmias), and better survival. These benefits are time-dependent: If coronary blood flow is reestablished within 1-2 hours of symptom onset, the relative risk of hospital death is reduced by 50%.

Non-ST-Elevation ACS (Chapters 6-10)

A. **Clinical Syndromes.** Unstable angina and non-ST-elevation MI.

B. **Prevalence.** Responsible for 1.5 million hospital admissions in United States each year; this number is expected to increase by 50% over the next 3 decades.

C. **Clinical Presentation.** Unstable angina can present as rest angina, new-onset severe angina, or increasing angina. Symptoms are similar to ST-elevation ACS (p. 4) and usually last less than 30 minutes. Atypical presentations—weakness, dyspnea, heart failure, dizziness—are more common in women, diabetics, and the elderly. Symptoms > 30 minutes in duration are often associated with elevated serum cardiac markers and acute

MI. Non-ST-elevation ACS can occur de novo or in patients with antecedent angina, and a precipitating factor is present in 50%. Up to 20% of infarcts go unrecognized by the physician or patient.

D. Classification. Patients are initially divided into risk categories (high- , intermediate- , or low-risk of short-term death or MI) based on clinical presentation, ECG, and serum cardiac markers (Table 6.2 p. 62). Risk stratification can identify patients most likely to benefit from GP IIb/IIIa inhibitors and the early invasive approach to management. Acute infarction/ ischemia is classified according to location and by the presence of associated mechanical, ischemic, or electrical complications (e.g., acute inferior ischemia complicated by Mobitz Type II 2° AV block and hypotension).

E. Electrocardiogram. The ECG can show transient ST-segment elevation with rapid resolution, ischemic ST-segment depression, T-wave inversion, nonspecific ST-T changes, or no changes at all. Evolution to Q-wave MI is uncommon (~ 25%).

F. Pathophysiology. The most common cause of non-ST-elevation ACS is microvascular embolization of platelet aggregates from nonocclusive thrombus at the site of plaque rupture. In contrast to ST-elevation MI, total occlusion of an epicardial coronary artery by clot is less common, myocardial necrosis is less extensive, and Q-waves develop in a minority of cases. Symptoms in unstable angina are due to transient reductions in coronary blood flow caused by periodic thrombosis and dynamic vasoconstriction from platelet activation and endothelial dysfunction. Occlusive thrombus is present in 10-20% in unstable angina, 20-40% in non-ST-elevation MI, and more than 80% in ST-elevation MI. Compared to ST-elevation MI, non-ST-elevation MI is associated with more spontaneous reperfusion, better collaterals, older age, and greater comorbidity (prior MI, multivessel disease, hypertension, heart failure, diabetes mellitus, peripheral vascular disease).

G. Management (Figure 7.1, p. 64). Initial therapy depends on the risk category of the patient. High-risk patients are best treated with an invasive strategy plus a GP IIb/IIIa inhibitor. Intermediate-risk patients are treated with antithrombin therapy with or without a GP IIb/IIIa inhibitor and/or an invasive strategy. Low-risk patients are treated medically, often as outpatients, in a manner similar to patients with chronic stable angina. Hospitalized patients without contraindications should also receive aspirin, beta-blockers, nitrates, antithrombin therapy, and cardiac monitoring. Clopidogrel and GP IIb/IIIa inhibitor use is complex (see pp. 77-78). Patients initially treated medically should be triaged to PCI for second positive troponin or ECG at 4-6 hours, recurrent ischemia, LV dysfunction (EF < 0.40), prior PCI or CABG, or a high-risk finding on stress testing. Fibrinolytics should be avoided in non-ST-elevation ACS due to the lack of clinical benefit and possible detrimental effect.

H. Prognosis

    1. **Unstable angina.** Prior to the availability of potent antiplatelet and antithrombin regimens and contemporary interventional techniques, medical therapy for unstable angina was associated with hospital mortality in 1-4% and nonfatal MI in 7-9% at 4-6 weeks. At 1 year, cardiac death occurred in 8-18%, nonfatal MI in 14-22%, and repeat hospitalization in 28-40%. Early use of clopidogrel, GP IIb/IIIa inhibitors, enoxaparin, and the early invasive strategy has improved clinical outcomes, although patients still remain at increased risk for adverse cardiac events.

    2. **Non-ST-elevation MI.** Compared to ST-elevation MI, non-ST-elevation MI is associated with smaller infarcts, better preservation of LV function, and lower in-hospital mortality. However, since non-ST-elevation MI is often associated with high-grade nonocclusive stenosis of the infarct-related artery, residual viable myocardium, and multivessel disease, reinfarction rates are higher and, by 1 year, mortality rates are similar.

Table 1.1. Clinical Features of Acute Coronary Syndromes

Feature	ST-Elevation ACS	Non-ST-Elevation ACS
Clinical syndromes	ST-elevation MI	Unstable angina; non-ST-elevation MI
Prevalence (U.S.)	600,000 cases per year	1.5 million cases per year
Presentation	Typical chest, neck, or jaw discomfort (pressure, burning, squeezing) lasting > 30 minutes. Atypical symptoms (weakness, dizziness, dyspnea) are more common in women, diabetics, and the elderly. Acute MI is silent in 20%, most often in diabetics with autonomic dysfunction	Same as ST-elevation ACS. Early risk stratification is important for prognosis and therapy (Chapters 6,7)
ECG	ST elevation ≥ 1 mm in at least 2 consecutive leads. LBBB and posterior MI are treated the same as ST-elevation ACS. Q-waves develop in 80% without reperfusion	ST depression > 0.5 mm and/or T wave inversion > 2.0 mm indicate high risk. Nonspecific ST-T changes or a normal ECG can be present. Complete coronary occlusion with ST-elevation develop in some during hospitalization. Q-waves develop in 20%
Pathophysiology	Plaque rupture with occlusive thrombus. Most ruptures develop in moderate stenoses with soft, lipid-rich cores and thin fibrous caps. Complete coronary occlusion develops in 90%	Plaque rupture with microvascular embolization of platelet aggregates from nonocclusive thrombus in most. Complete coronary occlusion develops in 10-40%. Intermittent thrombosis and dynamic vasoconstriction cause symptoms in unstable angina

Table 1.1. Clinical Features of Acute Coronary Syndromes (cont'd)

Feature	ST-Elevation ACS	Non-ST-Elevation ACS
Initial therapy	Primary PCI with stents. Fibrinolytic therapy if a cath lab with a skilled interventionalist and team is not available in a timely fashion	PCI with stents plus antithrombin therapy and a GP IIb/IIIa inhibitor for high-risk and some intermediate-risk patients. Antithrombin therapy for all other hospitalized patients followed by cath/PCI for recurrent ischemia or high-risk findings on noninvasive testing
Prognosis	Acute mortality 25-30%. In-hospital survival depends on speed and adequacy of reperfusion	In-hospital MI or death in unstable angina varies from 1-5%, depending on risk class. Non-ST-elevation MI has lower hospital mortality than ST-elevation MI but similar 1-year mortality due to more late events

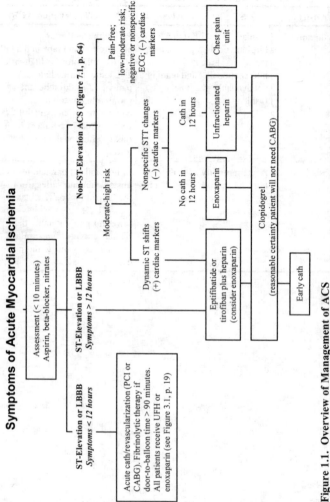

Figure 1.1. Overview of Management of ACS

(−) = negative, (+) = positive, ACS = acute coronary syndromes, CABG = coronary artery bypass grafting, ECG = electrocardiogram, LBBB = left bundle branch block, PCI = percutaneous coronary intervention, UFH = unfractionated heparin

ST-ELEVATION ACS

Chapter 2. Diagnosis and Evaluation 12

Chapter 3. Overview of Management 18

Chapter 4. Interventional Management 33

Chapter 5. Fibrinolytic Therapy 40

Chapter 2

Diagnosis and Evaluation of ST-Elevation ACS

Diagnosis

The diagnosis of acute MI requires one of two criteria. The first criterion requires the rise and fall of cardiac markers (troponin or CK-MB) *plus* one of the following: symptoms of ischemia, Q waves or ischemic changes on ECG, or coronary intervention. The second criterion is pathological findings indicative of acute MI.[1] There are important limitations to these criteria: acute MI can present with atypical symptoms, noncardiac disorders can manifest ischemic-type chest pain and ST-segment changes, and the rise and fall in cardiac markers is time-dependent and can be missed.

Symptoms

A. **Typical Presentation.** The most common presentation for acute MI is chest, neck, or jaw discomfort, which is usually described as a pressure, burning, or squeezing sensation lasting 30 minutes or longer. It is important to consider non-ischemic causes of chest pain at presentation—aortic dissection, pneumothorax, pericarditis, pulmonary embolus, esophageal rupture, ischemia/rupture of an intraabdominal organ— as these conditions can progress to life-threatening situations without expedient diagnosis and treatment.

B. **Atypical Presentations.** Weakness, dyspnea, heart failure, dizziness, and syncope are more common in diabetics and the elderly, and it is not uncommon for women to present with shortness of breath, fatigue, or jaw pain, stretched out over hours, rather than minutes.[1a] Pleuritic-type symptoms and pain reproduced by palpation are very unusual symptoms but do not exclude the possibility of acute MI.[2,3]

C. **Silent MI.** Up to 20% of infarcts are silent or go unrecognized,[4,5] most often in diabetics with autonomic dysfunction.

Electrocardiogram

A. **ST-Segment Shifts (Figure 2.1).** ST-elevation ≥ 1 mm in 2 or more contiguous leads (anterior, inferior, lateral) is required for the diagnosis of ST-elevation ACS. ST-elevation is usually convex ("out-pouching") in configuration and can persist from 48 hours to several weeks. Non-ischemic causes of ST-elevation can mimic acute MI on ECG, and these "pseudoinfarct" patterns can be seen in acute pericarditis, myocarditis, severe hyperkalemia, ventricular aneurysm, acute CNS disorder, left ventricular hypertrophy, Wolff-Parkinson-White syndrome, early repolarization, and apical hypertrophic cardiomyopathy.

B. **Evolution of ECG (Figure 2.1).**[6] Repolarization abnormalities evolve in a relatively predictable fashion. Marked, symmetrical peaking of the T wave ("hyperacute T waves") in the infarct region is the earliest finding in acute MI, but is often missed since it occurs very early (< 15 minutes) and resolves quickly. ECGs with hyperacute T waves should be repeated in 15 minutes to identify ST-elevation while preparing for fibrinolytic therapy or direct PCI. If transmural ischemia persists for more than a few minutes, peaked T waves evolve into convex ST segment elevation, which usually subsides in a few days but can last from hours to weeks. Infarct size and prognosis correlate with the number of ECG leads demonstrating ST-elevation. As acute MI continues to evolve, ST-elevation decreases and T waves begin to invert. The T waves usually deepen as the ST segments return to baseline, and T wave inversion can persist indefinitely or regress/disappear in months to years. Abnormal Q waves develop within hours to days of acute MI, usually while ST segments are still elevated, and persist indefinitely in 60-80%.

C. **Left Bundle Branch Block (LBBB) (p. 123).** Patients with acute MI and presumably new LBBB have high (20-25%) in-hospital mortality rates and derive substantial benefit from reperfusion therapy—a 21% reduction in death at 35 days (18.7% vs. 23.6%), which translates into 49 lives saved for every 1000 patients treated.[7] Nevertheless, patients with LBBB are up to 78% less likely to receive reperfusion therapy than those with ST-elevation.[8] Patients with acute MI and LBBB should undergo primary PCI if it is readily available; if not, they should be considered for fibrinolytic therapy.

Although the diagnosis of acute MI in the presence of LBBB is primarily based on history, 3 criteria that make acute MI more likely in the setting of LBBB: (1) ST-segment elevation $\geq$ 1 mm concordant with (in the same direction as) the major deflection of the QRS complex; (2) ST-segment depression $\geq$ 1 mm in lead V_1, V_2, or V_3; and (3) ST-segment elevation $\geq$ 5 mm discordant with (in the opposite direction to) the major deflection of the QRS complex.

D. Posterior MI. Posterior MI from left circumflex coronary artery occlusion presents with dominant R-waves and horizontal ST-segment depression $\geq$ 2 mm in the anterior precordial leads (V_1-V_2) and benefits from reperfusion therapy. Posterior infarction is often associated with acute inferior or inferolateral MI but can occur in isolation. ST-elevation in posterior chest leads V_{7-9} may improve the detection of posterior MI in patients with normal or nonspecific ECG changes.[9] Leads V_{7-9} are placed in the same horizontal plane as lead V_6 at the posterior axillary line, scapular angle, and paravertebral line, respectively.

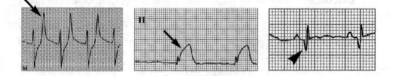

Figure 2.1. Evolution of ECG in ST-Elevation MI

Left panel: Hyperacute T waves (transient; may be missed).
Middle panel: Concave upward ST-segment elevation.
Right panel: Abnormal Q waves (develop in 80% without reperfusion).

E. **Paced Rhythm.** If acute MI is suspected in a patient with a pacemaker, the pacemaker can be temporarily reprogrammed to a lower rate to allow the intrinsic rhythm to be observed. ST-elevation is an indication for reperfusion therapy, although pacemaker-induced repolarization abnormalities can persist and mimic myocardial ischemia.

F. **Normal ECG.** Patients with symptoms of acute MI and a normal or nonspecific ECG should be managed as non-ST-elevation ACS (Chapter 7), unless posterior chest leads detect true posterior MI, in which case reperfusion therapy is indicated.

Serum Cardiac Markers

Several biochemical markers of myocardial necrosis can be used to establish the diagnosis of acute MI and estimate prognosis. No single cardiac marker is ideal, and each has its own advantages and disadvantages (Tables 2.1, 2.2). Since cardiac markers may not turn positive for hours, early treatment should be based on clinical presentation and initial ECG.

A. **Creatine Kinase.**[10-13] Enzyme levels usually exceed normal range by 6-10 hours and return to normal by 36-72 hours after acute MI. Levels should be obtained every 6-8 hours, and at least 3 negative values are required to rule out acute MI. CK-MB levels should be ≥ 3% of total creatine kinase levels in acute MI. Small infarcts can present with elevated cardiac troponin but normal CK-MB levels.[14]

B. **Cardiac Troponins (T/I).** These cardiac-specific regulatory proteins usually exceed normal range by 6-8 hours and remain elevated for 10-14 days after acute MI. Cardiac troponins are particularly useful to detect small MI, remote MI (> 24-48 hours), or acute MI in patients with skeletal muscle injury. At least 2 measurements should be obtained at 4-8 hour intervals. In non-ST-elevation ACS, elevated levels indicate increased risk of death or MI and identify patients most likely to benefit from GP IIb/IIIa inhibitors and the early invasive approach to management (Chapter 3).[15-22]

C. **Myoglobin.** This oxygen-binding heme protein is rapidly released after myocyte injury. Levels rise before CK-MB or troponins, but elevated levels can also be seen in skeletal muscle trauma, CPR, and renal failure. Elevated myoglobin levels are insufficient for the diagnosis of acute MI and require confirmation by CK-MB or cardiac troponins.[23,24] A negative value early after symptom onset is useful for ruling out acute MI.

Table 2.1. Serum Cardiac Markers

	CK-MB	Myoglobin	Cardiac Troponins
Description	High-energy transfer cytoplasmic protein	O_2-binding heme protein; rapidly released after myocyte injury	Regulatory proteins for calcium-dependent interactions between actin and myosin
Origin	Cardiac and skeletal muscle	Cardiac and skeletal muscle	Cardiac muscle
Release kinetics *Peak rise*	20 hours; sensitivity 94% at 8 hours and < 50% at 2 hours	2-3 hours	14 hours and 3-5 days (biphasic release)
Return to normal	36-72 hours	8-10 hours	10-14 days
Advantages	Able to detect early reinfarction	Best marker to detect very early MI	More sensitive and specific than CK-MB. Best marker for MI with skeletal muscle injury, small MI, or late MI (> 2-3 days)
Disadvantages	Low sensitivity for detection of very early (< 6 hr) MI, late (> 36 hr) MI, small MI; false-positive with skeletal muscle trauma, CPR, cardioversion, cardiac surgery	Low sensitivity for detection of late MI; false-positive with skeletal muscle trauma, CPR, renal failure	Low sensitivity for detection of early (< 6 hr) MI or late reinfarction

Table 2.1. Serum Cardiac Markers (cont'd)

	CK-MB	**Myoglobin**	**Cardiac Troponins**
Comments	Should be ≥ 3% of total CK in acute MI. With skeletal muscle injury, ratio of CK-MB mass to CK activity ≥ 2.5 suggests myocardial source of elevated CK-MB	Normal value useful for excluding early (4-8 hr) MI. Elevated levels insufficient to diagnose acute MI without elevated CK-MB or troponin levels	Identifies high-risk non-ST-elevation ACS and helps guide therapy. 30% of ACS patients with negative CK-MB have elevated troponins

Adapted from reference 128.

Table 2.2. Use of Serum Cardiac Markers

Subset	CK-MB	CK-MB Isoforms	Myoglobin	Cardiac Troponins
MI < 4 hours	–	–	+	–
MI 4-12 hours	+	+	+	+
MI > 2-10 days	–	–	–	±
Early reinfarction	+	+	±	–
Small MI	–	–	–	+
MI after operation or trauma	–	±	–	+

+ useful; ± some value; – not useful

Chapter 3
Overview of Management of ST-Elevation MI

Reperfusion Therapy (Figure 3.1)

It is now well-established that early reperfusion therapy with direct PCI or fibrinolysis reduces infarct size, preserves LV function, and improves survival in patients with acute MI < 12 hours and ST-elevation or presumably new LBBB on initial ECG. Nevertheless, only 70% of eligible patients in the GRACE[25] and NRMI Registries[26] received reperfusion therapy. Common reasons for withholding therapy included advanced age, absence of chest pain, left bundle branch block, history of heart failure, or prior MI/CABG surgery.

A. **Fibrinolytic Therapy (see pp. 40-51).** Following plaque rupture, circulating blood is exposed to highly thrombogenic constituents of the vessel wall (e.g., tissue factor, cholesterol esters), which rapidly induce intravascular thrombosis via activation of primary and secondary hemostasis (Figures 3.2, 3.3).[27-29] Primary hemostasis results in the formation of loosely adherent platelet aggregates at the site of plaque rupture; secondary hemostasis results in the formation of cross-linked fibrin (via activation of the coagulation cascade), which reinforces the primary hemostatic plug to produce fresh clot. By converting plasminogen into plasmin, fibrinolytic agents degrade the fibrin polymer to restore coronary perfusion.[30,31] For every 1000 patients treated with fibrinolytic therapy, approximately 20 lives are saved at 6 weeks.[7] Furthermore, these benefits are long-lasting: in the 10-year follow-up of GISSI-I, 18 lives were saved for every 1000 patients treated with streptokinase.[33] Survival benefit is apparent across all subgroups, regardless of age, gender, or comorbid medical conditions, but the greatest benefit is derived by patients who receive therapy in the first few hours and those at high risk (e.g., heart failure, LBBB). Despite the benefits of fibrinolytic therapy, important limitations exist: acute patency rates ≤ 80%, life-threatening intracranial bleeding in 0.5-1.5%, recurrent ischemia in 15-30%, and limited patient eligibility.[34]

Acute MI (ST-Elevation[1] or LBBB[2])[3]

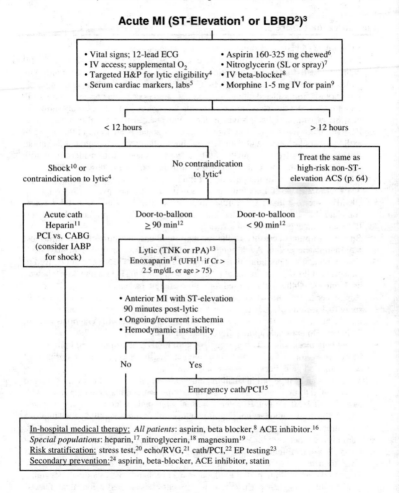

- Vital signs; 12-lead ECG
- IV access; supplemental O_2
- Targeted H&P for lytic eligibility[4]
- Serum cardiac markers, labs[5]
- Aspirin 160-325 mg chewed[6]
- Nitroglycerin (SL or spray)[7]
- IV beta-blocker[8]
- Morphine 1-5 mg IV for pain[9]

< 12 hours

> 12 hours

Shock[10] or contraindication to lytic[4]

No contraindication to lytic[4]

Treat the same as high-risk non-ST-elevation ACS (p. 64)

Acute cath
Heparin[11]
PCI vs. CABG
(consider IABP for shock)

Door-to-balloon ≥ 90 min[12]

Door-to-balloon < 90 min[12]

Lytic (TNK or rPA)[13]
Enoxaparin[14] (UFH[11] if Cr > 2.5 mg/dL or age > 75)

- Anterior MI with ST-elevation 90 minutes post-lytic
- Ongoing/recurrent ischemia
- Hemodynamic instability

No   Yes

Emergency cath/PCI[15]

In-hospital medical therapy: *All patients*: aspirin, beta blocker,[8] ACE inhibitor.[16]
Special populations: heparin,[17] nitroglycerin,[18] magnesium[19]
Risk stratification: stress test,[20] echo/RVG,[21] cath/PCI,[22] EP testing[23]
Secondary prevention:[24] aspirin, beta-blocker, ACE inhibitor, statin

Figure 3.1. Management of ST-Elevation MI

See footnotes, next page.

Footnotes for Figure 3.1.

1. ST-segment elevation ≥ 1 mm in 2 or more contiguous leads.
2. LBBB limits the ability to detect ST-elevation. Substantial mortality benefit for MI with new LBBB treated with fibrinolytics or PCI within 12 hours. Mortality rate without reperfusion therapy is high (~ 25%).
3. Posterior MI from isolated circumflex coronary artery occlusion presents without ST-elevation but benefits from acute reperfusion therapy. A 12-lead ECG may show ST-depression with upright T waves in leads V_{1-2} but can be normal or nonspecific. Posterior chest leads V_{7-9}, placed at the same horizontal plane as V_6 at the posterior axillary, scapular angle, and paravertebral lines, often show ST-segment elevation. Paced ventricular rhythms limit the ability to detect ST-elevation. Consider temporarily reprogramming the pacemaker below the intrinsic heart rate to observe ST-segment shifts, and treat with fibrinolytics or PCI if ST-segment elevation is present.
4. See Table 5.2 (p. 43) for contraindications to fibrinolytic therapy.
5. CK-MB every 6-8 hours x 3, cardiac troponins repeated at least once at 4-8 hours, complete blood count, platelet count, fibrinogen, lipid profile, electrolytes, BUN/creatinine, portable chest x-ray.
6. Buccal absorption of crushed or chewed nonenteric-coated aspirin produces the most rapid antiplatelet effects. Avoid enteric-coated preparations acutely due to delays in GI absorption and platelet inhibition. An aspirin suppository (325 mg) can be given to patients unable to take oral medications. Clopidogrel 300 mg PO loading dose followed by 75 mg PO q24h should be used for aspirin-allergic patients.
7. Administer up to 3 nitroglycerin tablets (0.4 mg) or 3 metered doses of nitroglycerin spray (0.4 mg) onto/under tongue at 5-minute intervals. Avoid if systolic BP < 90 mmHg, heart rate < 50 bpm, suspected RV infarction, or sildenafil (Viagra) use within 24 hours. Do not shake spray (affects metered dose).
8. Avoid beta-blocker acutely if systolic BP < 90 mmHg, heart rate < 50 bpm, severe heart failure, or history of significant bronchospasm. See p. 151 for dosing and administration guidelines.
9. Morphine can be repeated in small increments. Avoid in severe chronic lung disease (increased risk of respiratory depression). Hypoventilation can be reversed with naloxone (0.4-2.0 mg IV). Hypotension usually responds to leg elevation ± IV saline (200-300 cc if no pulmonary congestion). Bradycardia, nausea, vomiting often improve with atropine (0.5-1.0 mg IV).
10. Cardiogenic shock complicates 5-7% of acute infarctions, usually within the first few hours. Treatment requires immediate angiography, IABP counterpulsation, and revascularization, especially for patients < 75 years. Supportive measures include IV fluids to optimize filling pressures, dobutamine to enhance cardiac output, dopamine to maintain vital organ perfusion, and treatment of associated mechanical defects, arrhythmias, and conduction disturbances. A left ventricular assist device (LVAD) may be required as a stabilizing bridge to revascularization. It is important to exclude hypovolemia, RV infarction, papillary muscle rupture, ventricular septal defect, cardiac tamponade.

Footnotes for Figure 3.1. (cont'd)

11. Weight-adjusted IV heparin bolus of 60-70 U/kg (max. 5000 units) followed by initial heparin infusion of 12-15 U/kg/hr (max. 1000 U/hr) adjusted to aPTT 1.5-2.5 x control (50-75 seconds). May not be required in low-risk patients receiving streptokinase. For cath/PCI without GP IIb/IIIa inhibitor, give 60-100 U/kg IV bolus to achieve intraprocedural ACT of 300-350 seconds. For cath/PCI with GP IIb/IIIa inhibitor, give 60 U/kg IV bolus dose to achieve intraprocedural ACT of 200-250 seconds.

12. Interventionalist performs > 75 cases per year. If skilled interventionalist is not available, consider transfer to interventional center for emergency PCI as long as first door-to-balloon time can be within 90-100 minutes.

13. TNK-tPA is administered as a single, weight-adjusted IV bolus over 5 seconds: < 60 kg (30 mg); 60-69 kg (35 mg); 70-79 kg (40 mg); 80-89 kg (45 mg); ≥ 90 kg (50 mg). rPA is administered as a 10 U IV bolus over 2 minutes, repeated in 30 minutes x 1. See table 5.3 (pp. 45-46) for other fibrinolytic regimens.

14. Enoxaparin dose: 1 mg/kg SQ q12h x 2-8 days (optimal duration unknown). Consider initial bolus of 30 mg IV (ASSENT trial).

15. Primary stenting is preferred over primary PTCA. Clopidogrel 300 mg PO loading dose is recommended prior to stenting, followed by 75 mg PO q24h x 1 year. Routine use of a GP IIb/IIIa inhibitor is reasonable (see Table 9.3, p. 83 for dose). When a GP IIb/IIIa inhibitor is used, an initial UFH IV bolus of 60 U/kg is recommended to achieve an intraprocedural ACT of 200-250 seconds. When no GP IIb/IIIa inhibitor is used, an initial UFH IV bolus of 60-100 U/kg is recommended to achieve an intraprocedural ACT of 300-350 seconds. Patients with 1- or 2-vessel disease and successful PCI can be considered for discharge on day 3 if age < 70 yrs and EF > 45%.

16. Start oral ACE inhibitor at low dose as soon as patient is stabilized from MI (after reperfusion and once blood pressure has stabilized; usually no sooner than 6 hours). Titrate upward over 24-48 hours, as tolerated. See p. 148 for dosing and administration guidelines. Continue indefinitely if ejection fraction is reduced. For uncomplicated MI without LV dysfunction, discontinue after 4-6 weeks or consider long-term therapy for secondary prevention.

17. In addition to use with acute reperfusion therapy, IV heparin (aPTT 50-75 seconds) is indicated for recurrent ischemia or reinfarction and for patients at high risk of thromboembolism (e.g., large anterior MI, previous embolus, atrial fibrillation, possibly LV thrombus). Subcutaneous heparin 5000-7000 U q12h or enoxaparin 1 mg/kg q12h should be considered in others during periods of prolonged immobilization.

18. IV nitroglycerin is continued x 24-48 hours for large anterior MI, heart failure, hypertension, or recurrent ischemia. Tachyphylaxis can develop as early as 24 hours after continuous therapy and may require an increase in dose or a 12-hour nitrate-free interval.

19. Magnesium (1-2 gm IV) is indicated for hypomagnesemia or torsade de pointes.

20. Either of two stress testing approaches is acceptable: (1) submaximal stress test at 4-7

Footnotes for Figure 3.1. (cont'd)

days followed by a symptom-limited stress test at 6 weeks; or (2) symptom-limited stress test at 10-14 days.

21. Echo/RVG is recommended for large MI, prior MI, heart failure, sustained hypotension, murmur, pericarditis, suspected LV dysfunction, or mechanical complication.

22. Cardiac catheterization is recommended for spontaneous or inducible ischemia, heart failure, EF < 40%, prior revascularization, VT or VF > 48 hours post-MI.

23. EP testing is recommended for VT or VF > 2 days from MI.

24. Secondary prevention measures include aspirin, beta-blocker, ACE inhibitor, statin, exercise, smoking cessation, weight control, Mediterranean diet. Consider gemfibrozil, niacin, and/or fish oil (omega-3 fatty acids) for low HDL cholesterol. Control hypertension (blood pressure ≤ 130/85 mmHg), diabetes mellitus (HgbA1c < 7%), and dyslipidemia (LDL cholesterol ≤ 100 mg/dL; HDL-cholesterol > 40 mg/dL; triglyceride ≤ 150 mg/dL). Provide instructions to patient and family on the use of nitrates for recurrent pain, when to return to the emergency room, the purpose and dose of each discharge medication, and the importance of compliance.

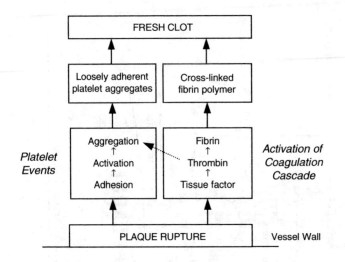

Figure 3.2. Pathophysiology of Acute Coronary Syndromes

Intravascular thrombosis is central to the pathogenesis of ACS. Plaque rupture exposes circulating blood to vessel wall contents, which rapidly induce clot formation via activation of two complementary systems: platelets and the coagulation cascade. Abrupt, occlusive, intracoronary thrombosis manifests clinically as acute ST-elevation MI; nonocclusive thrombosis presents as unstable angina or non-ST-elevation MI. The amount of angiographic thrombus has been correlated with the severity of clinical presentation. Numerous phospholipids, glycoproteins, enzymes, and other factors are involved in this process (Figure 3.3).

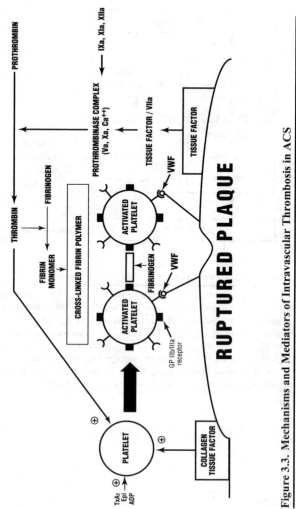

Figure 3.3. Mechanisms and Mediators of Intravascular Thrombosis in ACS

See footnotes, next page.

Footnotes for Figure 3.3.

Plaque rupture exposes the highly thrombogenic lipid-rich core to circulating blood, resulting in activation of primary and secondary hemostasis.

Primary hemostasis (platelet plug formation): Plaque rupture induces platelets to proceed through adhesion, activation, and aggregation. <u>Platelet adhesion</u>: Initiated by the binding of von Willebrand factor (vWF), an adhesive glycoprotein released from the injured vessel wall, to the platelet glycoprotein (GP) Ib receptor. <u>Platelet activation</u>: Platelets are exposed to multiple agonists at the same time (e.g., ADP, thromboxane A_2, epinephrine, thrombin), which triggers a series of events within the platelet, including increased cytosolic calcium, cell shape changes, phosphorylation of proteins, release of granules and lysosomes, arachidonic acid metabolism, and conformational change in the GP IIb/IIIa receptor complex so that it becomes expressed and active on the platelet surface. <u>Platelet aggregation</u>: 50,000-80,000 GP IIb/IIIa receptors reside on the surface of activated platelets. Fibrinogen is the most important ligand of the GP IIb/IIIa receptor and can bind two GP IIb/IIIa receptors simultaneously, creating a molecular platelet-to-platelet bridge.

Secondary hemostasis (fibrin formation): The principal mechanism for thrombin generation and fibrin deposition following plaque rupture is exposure of tissue factor, a low-molecular-weight glycoprotein concentrated in vessel wall macrophages and vulnerable plaques. Tissue factor initiates the extrinsic pathway of coagulation by forming a high-affinity complex with clotting factors VII/VIIa. Thrombin plays a critical role in clot formation: it converts fibrinogen to fibrin, activates clotting factors V and VIII and protein C, and is a potent stimulus for platelet activation and aggregation. The formation and polymerization of fibrin is crucial to clot stabilization and propagation, converting the unstable primary platelet plug into an adherent "red" thrombus.

B. Percutaneous Coronary Intervention (PCI) (Figure 3.4 and pp. 33-38).
To overcome the deficiencies of fibrinolytic therapy, emergency PCI is
being used in many institutions to achieve acute reperfusion. Advantages of
primary PCI in the hands of experienced interventionalists (> 75 cases per
year) at high-volume centers (> 200-300 cases per year) include high (85-
95%) infarct vessel patency rates; low rates of recurrent ischemia,
reinfarction, death, and stroke; avoidance of intracranial bleeding; shortened
length of hospital stay; and the ability to treat lytic-ineligible patients.[34]

C. PTCA vs. Fibrinolysis. Ten randomized trials were performed in 2606
patients through 1997 comparing primary PTCA to either streptokinase (4
studies), 3-4–hour tPA regimens (3 studies), or accelerated tPA (3
studies).[35-42] A meta-analysis of these trials demonstrated marked benefits
for PTCA, including 30-50% reductions in death, reinfarction, and stroke
at 30 days and 6 months and virtual elimination of intracranial bleeding
(0.1% vs. 1.1%) (Table 3.1).[34] It was estimated that 21 lives would be saved
at 30 days for every 1000 patients treated with PCI instead of fibrinolytic
therapy (mortality rate 4.4% vs. 6.5%). High-risk patients (age > 70,
anterior MI, heart rate > 100, Killip class > 1) had the greatest reductions in
death and stroke (Table 3.2), but even low-risk patients had less recurrent
ischemia/reinfarction and shorter hospital stays. In a pooled analysis of
2635 patients enrolled in 10 randomized trials of primary angioplasty vs.
fibrinolytic therapy, primary angioplasty reduced the 30-day risk of death,
reinfarction, and stroke by 54% in patients presenting within 2 hours of
symptom onset (5.8% vs. 12.5%), by 39% at 2-4 hours (8.6% vs. 14.2%),
and by 61% after 4 hours (7.7% vs. 19.6%).[43] Major adverse cardiac events
increased with increasing time to presentation for fibrinolytic therapy but
not for angioplasty. In the National Registry of Myocardial Infarction
(NRMI), which compared primary PTCA to fibrinolytic therapy in > 62,000
patients, PTCA was associated with 37% lower mortality at high-volume
interventional centers but had no impact on survival at low-volume
hospitals.[44] Nevertheless, PTCA reduced the risk of stroke by 64% (0.4%
vs. 1.1%) at high- and low-volume hospitals. These results support the
superiority of primary PTCA over fibrinolytic therapy for reducing death,
reinfarction, stroke, and intracranial hemorrhage when skilled personnel and
adequate equipment are available in a timely fashion.

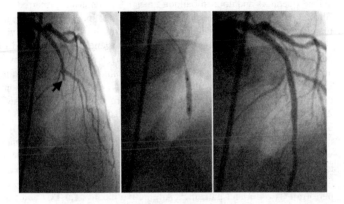

Figure 3.4. Primary Stenting for Acute MI

Left panel: Total occlusion of left anterior descending (LAD) coronary artery (arrow) resulting in acute ST-elevation MI.
Middle panel: Balloon-expandable stent.
Right panel: Final result demonstrating no residual stenosis.

D. PTCA vs. Stents. In a meta-analysis of 2844 patients in 8 randomized trials of PTCA vs. stents for acute MI, the composite endpoint of death, reinfarction, and target vessel revascularization was reduced by 46% at 6 months with stents (14% vs. 26%, p < 0.0001).[45] In CADILLAC, the largest of the randomized trials, stents reduced the rate of clinical and angiographic restenosis by ~ 50% (Table 4.2, p. 35).[46] These data support the superiority of stents over PTCA (although the entire benefit is in reduction of restenosis; no effect on death or MI has yet been shown) and indicate that primary stenting should be considered the routine reperfusion strategy for acute MI.

E. Recommendations (Figure 3.1 and pp. 30-39). Primary stenting with skilled operators and door-to-balloon times < 90 minutes is preferred over fibrinolytic therapy for ST-elevation MI. If a skilled interventionalist is not readily available, recommendations are based on lytic eligibility. Lytic-eligible patients should be given a fibrinolytic agent, then transferred for emergency PCI for ongoing or recurrent ischemia, labile hemodynamics, or anterior MI with persistent ST-elevation 90 minutes after lytic therapy. Lytic-ineligible patients should be rapidly transferred to an interventional center for PCI or CABG. If ongoing trials confirm the results of DANAMI-2 and PRAGUE (Table 5.1, p. 41), rapid hospital transfer to an interventional center for primary PCI may be preferred to on-site lytic therapy for patients who present to hospitals without PCI capabilities and with systems in place to assure rapid transfer. Another option is to leave treatment protocols in place, as recommended in the C-PORT trial, so that hospitals that lack on-site surgical backup could be trained and prepared to perform PCI on urgent patients.[32] Adjunctive medical for PCI and non-medical therapies are described on pages 36-38 and 97-103, respectively.

Table 3.1. Meta-analysis of 10 Randomized Trials of Primary PTCA vs. Fibrinolytic Therapy for ST-Elevation MI[34]*

	Primary PTCA (n = 1348)	Lytic Therapy (n = 1377)	p-Value
30-Day Outcomes (%)			
Mortality	4.4	6.5	0.02
Reinfarction	2.9	5.3	0.002
Stroke	0.7	1.9	0.02
Hemorrhagic stroke	0.1	1.1	0.01
6-Month Outcomes (%)			
Mortality	5.1	7.5	0.039
Reinfarction	4.2	8.4	0.0001
Death or MI	9.6	15.2	0.0001

* From the Primary Coronary Angioplasty Trialists (PCAT) Collaboration

Table 3.2. Primary PTCA vs. Fibrinolytic Therapy for ST-Elevation MI: Subgroup Analysis of 10 Randomized Trials[34]*

| Subgroup | 30-day Death or Reinfarction (%) | | Odds Ratio | Events Prevented per 1000 Patients |
	Primary PTCA (n = 1348)	Lytic Therapy (n = 1377)		
Age < 60 years	4.3	8.2	0.48	41
60-70 years	6.3	12.8	0.51	64
> 70 years	13.3	23.6	0.43	118
Male	5.7	12.2	0.53	61
Female	11.7	16.4	0.29	82
No diabetes	6.5	11.8	0.45	59
Diabetes	9.2	19.3	0.52	97
No prior MI	6.6	11.5	0.43	58
Prior MI	9.7	22.7	0.57	114
Non-anterior MI	6.2	12.0	0.48	60
Anterior MI	8.2	14.5	0.43	73

* From the Primary Coronary Angioplasty Trialists (PCAT) Collaboration

General Measures (Figure 3.1, Table 3.3)

A. Emergency Department. Initial management of ST-elevation MI includes administration of aspirin, nitrates, heparin, and beta-blockers, and rapid triage to PCI or fibrinolytic therapy. The evaluation process should be streamlined to obtain a "door-to-lytic" time within 30 minutes or a "door-to-balloon" time within 90 minutes. Initial assessment should also exclude the presence of a life-threatening condition that can mimic acute MI: aortic dissection, pulmonary embolism, acute pericarditis, pneumothorax, esophageal rupture, or ischemia/rupture of an intra-abdominal organ. Additional measures include IV line access, supplemental oxygen for respiratory distress or hypoxemia, morphine sulfate for analgesia, vasopressors and possibly intra-aortic balloon pump counterpulsation for hypotension or shock, and control of precipitating factors (e.g., anemia, hypoxemia, hypovolemia, hypotension, hyperthyroidism, infection).

B. Early Hospitalization. Over the first 24 hours of hospitalization, aspirin, heparin, and beta-blockers are continued, and analgesics and anti-anxiety medications are prescribed as needed. Once reperfusion has occurred and blood pressure has stabilized (usually no sooner than 6 hours), an oral ACE inhibitor is started at low dose and titrated upward. An ACE inhibitor is definitely indicated for clinical heart failure, left ventricular dysfunction, anterior MI, or hypertension; for LV ejection fraction > 45%, use of an ACE inhibitor is discretionary. IV nitroglycerin and magnesium are recommended for special patient populations (Table 3.4). Monitoring and other general measures include vital signs every 30 minutes until stable, then every 4 hours; pulse oximetry for at least one day; bed rest with bedside commode for 12 hours followed by a progressive increase in activity; NPO until pain free followed by a clear liquid diet and then a low saturated fat diet; and stool softeners.

C. Late Hospitalization (> 24 hours). Aspirin, beta-blockers, and ACE inhibitors (if started) are continued throughout hospitalization, and unfractionated or low-molecular-weight heparin is usually given for a total of 3-5 days or until revascularization. Early recognition and treatment of mechanical, ischemic, and electrical complications is critical (Chapters 13, 14). Predischarge risk stratification is used to identify residual ischemia, assess LV function, and identify patients at increased risk for malignant ventricular arrhythmias (Chapter 12).

D. Post-Discharge Measures. Emphasis is placed on secondary prevention through cardiac rehabilitation;[50,51] lifestyle modification (e.g., Mediterranean diet,[52,53] smoking cessation,[54] weight control, exercise[55]); treatment of hypertension (BP ≤ 130/85 mmHg),[56] dyslipidemia (LDL cholesterol < 100 mg/dL, HDL cholesterol > 40 mg/dL, triglyceride < 150 mg/dL),[57] and diabetes (Hgb A1$_C$ < 7%);[58] and use of aspirin,[59,60] beta-blockers,[61] statins,[62] and ACE inhibitors.[63,64]

Table. 3.3. Early Management of ST-Elevation MI in All Patients Without Contraindications

Treatment	Indications	Dosing and Administration
Aspirin	First dose of 162-325 mg of nonenteric-coated preparation chewed acutely, followed indefinitely by 75-325 mg (PO) q24h of an enteric or nonenteric preparation. A rectal suppository (325 mg) can be used for patients unable to take medications orally	pp. 75, 150
Nitrates	Sublingual nitroglycerin tablets (0.4 mg) or aerosol spray (0.5-1.0 seconds) every 5 minutes x 3 to control ischemic pain. Avoid in RV infarction, sildenafil (Viagra) use within 24 hours, severe hypotension, bradycardia, or tachycardia	p. 160
Beta-blockers	Started IV acutely, then switched to oral therapy	p. 151
ACE inhibitors	Started PO at low dose as soon as patient is stable (after reperfusion and once blood pressure has stabilized, usually no sooner than 6 hours post-MI), then titrated upward over 1-4 days, as tolerated. Definite for LV dysfunction; optional for preserved LV function. Ensure adequate hydration prior to initiating therapy	p. 148
Antithrombin therapy	Used as an adjunct to reperfusion therapy. May not be necessary with streptokinase unless at high risk for thromboembolism. Unfractionated heparin or low-molecular-weight heparin can be used	pp. 157-159
Reperfusion therapy	PCI with stenting is preferred over fibrinolytic therapy when a skilled interventionalist is available. Routine use of a GP IIb/IIIa inhibitor is reasonable	PCI (p. 33); fibrinolytics (p. 40)
Morphine	1-5 mg IV bolus over 1-5 minutes to control ischemic pain; can repeat every 5-30 minutes as needed. Also useful in heart failure	p. 160
Oxygen	1-4 L/min by nasal cannula for 2-3 hours is given by convention, but data to support its routine use are lacking. Higher doses by different delivery systems for longer durations may be required in hypoxemic patients to keep arterial oxygen saturation > 90%	p. 162

Table 3.4. Early Management of ST-Elevation MI in Special Patient Populations

Treatment	Indications	Dosing and Administration
Antiarrhythmics	Adenosine (p. 148), amiodarone (p. 149), atropine (p. 150), lidocaine (p. 159), magnesium sulfate (p. 160), procainamide (p. 162)	
Calcium antagonists	Rate-limiting calcium antagonist for patients with a contraindication to beta-blockers	p. 152
Dobutamine	Acute heart failure without shock or hemodynamically-significant RV infarction not responding to IV fluids	p. 154
Dopamine	Severe hypotension	p. 154
Epinephrine	Cardiac arrest; profound bradycardia or hypotension	p. 155
Furosemide	Acute treatment of pulmonary congestion associated with LV dysfunction	p. 156
GP IIb/IIIa inhibitors	Adjunct to PCI	p. 156
IABP counterpulsation	Cardiogenic shock; as a stabilizing bridge to PCI or surgery in critically ill patients	p. 99
Nitrates (IV)	Heart failure; ongoing or recurrent ischemia; possibly for large anterior MI. Data to support routine use beyond 24 hours are lacking	p. 160
Nitroprusside	Hypertensive emergencies; acute heart failure; afterload reduction for acute mitral/aortic regurgitation or acute ventricular septal defect	p. 162
Pacemaker	Prophylaxis against hemodynamic collapse in patients at high risk of progression to complete heart block; treatment of high-grade AV block or bradyarrhythmias not responding to atropine	p. 100

AV = atrio-ventricular, LV= left ventricular, PCI = percutaneous coronary intervention, RV = right ventricular

Chapter 4

Interventional Management of ST-Elevation MI

Primary Stenting vs. Balloon Angioplasty (PTCA)

A. Randomized Trials (Table 4.1). The efficacy and safety of primary stenting has been evaluated in several prospective randomized trials. In Stent-PAMI, 900 patients with acute MI were randomized to the Palmaz-Schatz heparin-coated stent or PTCA.[66] Primary stenting resulted in less recurrent ischemia and restenosis, but TIMI-3 flow rates were lower and 6-month mortality was higher in the stent group. More recently, 2082 patients with acute MI were randomized to MultiLink stenting or PTCA (with or without abciximab) in CADILLAC. In contrast to STENT-PAMI, stenting resulted in better event-free survival at 6 months due to less clinical and angiographic restenosis.[46] Abciximab reduced the rates of recurrent ischemia leading to early repeat target vessel revascularization after PTCA or stenting and, in a recent systematic overview of RAPPORT, ISAR-2, ADMIRAL, and CADILLAC, reduced the composite endpoint of death, MI, and revascularization at 6 months (Table 4.2).[66a] In a meta-analysis of 2844 patients in 8 randomized trials of PTCA vs. stenting for acute MI, the composite endpoint of death, reinfarction, and target vessel revascularization at 6 months was reduced by 46% with stents (14% vs. 26%, $p < 0.0001$).[45] Sirolimus- and paclitaxel-eluting stents have led to dramatic reductions in restenosis compared to standard stents (< 5% vs. 20-30%) (Table 4.3), but they have yet to be evaluated in the setting of ST-elevation MI. The role of stents vs. PTCA for culprit lesions in small (< 2.5 mm) diameter vessels and saphenous vein grafts awaits definition.

B. Recommendations. Primary stenting in conjunction with a GP IIb/IIIa inhibitor should be considered the routine reperfusion strategy for patients with acute ST-elevation MI, when available.

Table 4.1. Randomized Trials of Stenting vs. PTCA for Acute MI

Trial	N	Stent	Results (Stent vs. PTCA)
CADILLAC[46] (2002)	2082	MultiLink, MultiLink-Duet	Stents resulted in less clinical and angiographic restenosis but had no effect on death or MI. Abciximab prevented early thrombotic events but had no impact on restenosis
STOPAMI[70] (2002)	162	Stent + abciximab vs. tPA + abciximab	Compared to tPA, stents resulted in smaller infarct size ($p < 0.05$), better myocardial salvage ($p = 0.001$), and a trend toward less death or MI at 6 months (7.4% vs. 17.3%, $p = 0.053$)
STENTIM-2[71] (2000)	211	Wiktor	Stents resulted in less ARS (23.3% vs. 39.6%, $p < 0.05$) but no difference in procedural success, EFS, or TLR at 6 and 12 months
FRESCO[72] (2000)	150	GR	Stents resulted in less MACE (9% vs. 28%, $p < 0.01$) and ARS (17% vs. 43%, $p < 0.001$) at 6 months
STENT-PAMI[66] (1999)	900	HCPSS	Stents resulted in less TIMI-3 flow (89% vs. 93%, $p < 0.05$), less ischemic TVR at 6 months (7.7% vs. 17%, $p < 0.001$) and at 1 year (10.6% vs 21%, $p < 0.0001$), less ARS at 6 months (23% vs. 35%, $p < 0.001$), and less MACE (17% vs. 24.8%, $p < 0.01$), but higher mortality at 1 year (5.8% vs. 3.0%, $p = 0.054$)
PASTA[73] (1999)	136	PSS	Stents resulted in similar success (99% vs. 97%), less in-hospital MACE (6% vs. 19%, $p < 0.05$) and 1-year MACE (22% vs. 49%, $p < 0.001$), and less ARS at 6 months (17% vs. 37.5%, $p < 0.05$)

ARS = angiographic restenosis, EFS = event-free survival, GR = Gianturco Roubin, HCPPS = heparin-coated Palmaz-Schatz stent, TLR = target lesion revascularization, MACE = major adverse cardiac events

Table 4.2. Abciximab as Adjunct to PCI for Acute MI

| Trial | No. Patients | Death, Recurrent Infarction, or Any Target Vessel Revascularization at 6 Months | |
		Abciximab (%)	Placebo (%)
ADMIRAL	300	22.8	33.8
CADILLAC	2082	13.9	16.2
ISAR-2	401	11.9	17.5
RAPPORT	483	28.2	28.1
Combined	3266	16.6*	19.8

* OR 0.80, 95% CI: 0.67-0.97

Table 4.3. Recent Drug-Eluting Stent Trials for Coronary Disease

| Study | Design | Results (Drug-Eluting Stent vs. Standard Stent) | | |
		Late Loss	Restenosis	Clinical
RAVEL[81] (2002) (n = 238)	Sirolimus-eluting Bx Velocity stent vs. standard stent	– 0.01 mm vs. 0.80 mm (p < 0.001)	0% vs. 26% (p < 0.001); 0% vs. 47% in 44 diabetics (p = 0.002)	1-year MACE 5.8% vs. 28.8% (p < 0.001)
SIRIUS[82] (2002) (n = 400 of 1101)	Sirolimus-eluting Bx Velocity stent vs. standard stent	0.06 mm vs. 0.55 mm (p < 0.001)	2.0% vs. 31.1% at 8 months (p < 0.001)	9-month MACE 9.2% vs. 19.4% (p = 0.009)
ELUTES[83] (2002) (n = 192)	Paclitaxel-eluting V-Flex Plus stent without polymer (tested at 4 doses) vs. standard stent. Results presented for best dose	0.10 mm vs. 0.73 mm (p = 0.002)	3.1% vs. 20.6% (p = 0.055)	30-day MACE 1.1% for drug-stent; 1-year TLR 5% vs. 16%

Late loss = difference in minimum lumen diameter immediately after stenting and at follow-up (reflects degree of intimal thickening), MACE = major adverse cardiac events, MI = myocardial infarction, TLR = target lesion revascularization

Adjunctive Pharmacotherapy for PCI

A. **Preprocedural Pharmacotherapy ("Facilitated PCI").** The ability of
fibrinolytic therapy to restore early patency prior to primary PTCA was
evaluated in 606 patients with acute MI in PACT.[67] The administration of
tPA (50 mg IV bolus) immediately before angiography resulted in better
TIMI-3 flow prior to PTCA (33% vs. 15%, p < 0.001) with less need for
immediate intervention and no increase in bleeding complications, but
preprocedural tPA had no impact on coronary blood flow, LV function, or
clinical outcome after PCI. Compared to patients not receiving tPA prior to
hospital transport for urgent PCI in PRAGUE, administration of tPA prior
to transport resulted in a higher rate of death, reinfarction, or stroke at 30
days (15% vs. 8%).[49] The role for preprocedural ("upstream") low-dose
fibrinolytic therapy ± GP IIb/IIIa inhibitors is under investigation.

B. **Intraprocedural Pharmacotherapy**

1. **Aspirin and clopidogrel (pp. 75-78).** Prior to PCI, all patients should
receive 325 mg of nonenteric chewable aspirin followed by 75-325 mg
(PO) q24h long term. Patients undergoing stenting should also receive
clopidogrel 300 mg PO followed by 75 mg PO q24h for 1 year.[398]

2. **GP IIb/IIIa inhibitors (pp. 79-84).** Trials of abciximab as an adjunct
to primary PTCA (RAPPORT,[68] CADILLAC[46]) or stenting
(ADMIRAL,[69] CADILLAC) have demonstrated a reduction in events.
In a meta-analysis of 1738 patients in 3 randomized trials of abciximab
vs. placebo as adjuncts to stenting for acute MI (CADILLAC,
ADMIRAL, ISAR-2), the composite endpoint of death, reinfarction,
and target vessel revascularization at 6 months was reduced by 28%
with abciximab (12% vs. 16.6%, p < 0.001).[45] If abciximab is used, an
IV bolus of 0.25 mg/kg is given at the start of the procedure followed
by an IV infusion of 0.125 mcg/kg/min (max. 10 mcg/min) x 12 hours.
There are insufficient data to recommend eptifibatide or tirofiban as
adjuncts to PCI for ST-elevation MI.

3. **Heparin.** Unfractionated heparin is usually given as a weight-adjusted
IV bolus of 60-100 U/kg to achieve an intraprocedural ACT of 300-350
seconds. When abciximab is used, an IV heparin bolus of 60 U/kg is
recommended to achieve a target ACT of 200-250 seconds. Prolonged
heparin infusions following successful PCI are of no proven value. As

an alternative to unfractionated heparin, low-molecular-weight heparin may be easier to administer and associated with better clinical outcomes (ASSENT-3, p. 55), but further testing will be needed before it is adopted widely.

Procedural Technique

A. Technical Details. PTCA or stenting is performed on the infarct vessel to achieve a residual stenosis < 30% and TIMI-3 flow. Emergency PCI is usually limited to the culprit vessel, but multivessel intervention may be indicated for patients in cardiogenic shock. Intra-aortic balloon pump counterpulsation is often employed in patients with multivessel disease and ongoing ischemia, hypotension, pulmonary edema, or LV dysfunction. Following successful PCI, stable, low-risk patients can be managed in a step-down unit and can often be discharged on the third hospital day. Stress testing is not routinely performed after successful PCI.[74]

B. Deficiencies of PCI
   1. **Reperfusion arrhythmias**. Ventricular fibrillation and brady-arrhythmias are more common with right coronary artery (RCA) intervention. To minimize this risk, IV beta-blockers, low-osmolar ionic contrast, continuous monitoring of O_2 saturation, and adequate hydration are recommended prior to reperfusion of the RCA.
   2. **Bleeding complications.** Compared to fibrinolytic therapy, PCI is associated with less intracranial hemorrhage but more blood transfusions. Meticulous vascular access technique, monitoring of ACT levels, avoidance of post-procedural heparin, and early sheath removal are indicated to minimize bleeding complications. A target ACT of 200-250 seconds is recommended when abciximab is used.
   3. **Ischemic complications.** Recurrent ischemia occurs in 10-15% of patients following PCI, and early reocclusion increases hospital mortality by 3-fold. Stents reduce ischemic complications (3% after stents vs. 15% after balloon angioplasty vs. 30% after lytics) and early reinfarction (< 1% after stents vs. 1-2% after balloon angioplasty vs. 8% after lytics).[74]

Primary PCI for Cardiogenic Shock

Patients in cardiogenic shock are usually taken to the catheterization laboratory for hemodynamic stabilization with an intra-aortic balloon pump (IABP), angiography, and emergency revascularization. Nonrandomized studies reported survival rates of 40-86% after PTCA compared to 30% after lytic therapy and 10% after medical therapy.[75-78] In GUSTO-I, an aggressive revascularization strategy of PTCA or CABG was independently associated with improved survival at 30 days.[79] More recently, in the SHOCK trial, 302 patients were randomized to an early invasive approach of emergency catheterization followed by immediate revascularization (PTCA or CABG) or an early conservative approach of initial medical stabilization followed by revascularization for recurrent ischemia. Revascularization was performed in 87% of patients in the invasive group and 34% of patients in the conservative group. One-year survival was 46.7% in the early revascularization group and 33.6% in the initial medical stabilization group (p < 0.03); benefit was apparent only for patients < 75 years (survival 51.6% with early revascularization vs. 33.3% with initial medical therapy). At 1 year, 83% of survivors were in NYHA heart failure Class I or II.[80] These data support the use of immediate angiography, IABP counterpulsation, and emergency revascularization for cardiogenic shock, particularly in patients < 75 years old.

Coronary Artery Bypass Graft (CABG) Surgery

CABG is not widely utilized during acute MI due to logistical considerations and the general success of PCI as a therapy. However, CABG should be considered as part of an integrated revascularization strategy, especially for patients in cardiogenic shock. Indications for emergency CABG in the setting of acute MI are shown in Table 4.4.

Table 4.4. Indications for CABG in Acute MI

- Left main stenosis > 50% with left anterior descending or left circumflex coronary infarct vessel

- Left main stenosis > 75% with right coronary infarct vessel

- Severe proximal multivessel disease not suitable for PCI, especially if the infarct vessel is patent

- Severe multivessel disease with cardiogenic shock

- Failed mechanical reperfusion with infarct duration < 6-12 hours, a large area of jeopardized myocardium, and ongoing ischemic pain, especially in the presence of well-developed collaterals

Chapter 5

Fibrinolytic Therapy for ST-Elevation MI

If a skilled interventionalist is not available, patients with acute MI and ST-elevation or LBBB without contraindications should receive fibrinolytic therapy. Hospital transfer for emergency PCI after lytic therapy is recommended for ongoing or recurrent ischemia, labile hemodynamics, or anterior MI with persistent ST-elevation 90 minutes after lytic therapy. As an alternative to on-site lytic therapy, DANAMI-2 demonstrated the safety and efficacy of hospital transfer for primary PCI. Among 1129 patients with severe (≥ 4 mm ST-elevation) MI < 12 hours, hospital transfer resulted in a 40% reduction in the composite endpoint of death, reinfarction, and disabling stroke at 30 days compared to onsite lytic therapy (8.5% vs. 14.2%).[47] There were no deaths during hospital transfer, and time from door of first hospital to balloon inflation was only 100 minutes. Similar results were reported in the PRAGUE trials (Table 5.1). Larger trials are underway, including pilot studies of direct transfer to a PCI center, which may not necessarily be the nearest hospital.

Overview of Fibrinolytic Therapy

A. **Primary Goal of Therapy.** The primary goal of fibrinolytic therapy is to achieve early coronary and myocardial reperfusion, which reduces infarct size, preserves LV function, reduces the risk of arrhythmias and heart failure, and improves survival. Fibrinolytic agents differ with respect to side effects, cost, and degree of systemic fibrinolysis (pp. 45-46),[86] which determines the need for conjunctive heparin therapy. Acute (90-minute) patency rates differ among agents, but by 3 hours patency rates are similar. Until GUSTO-I was published in 1993, randomized trials suggested that all agents were equally effective at preserving LV function and reducing mortality. GUSTO-I showed that an accelerated tPA regimen (100 mg infused over 90 minutes) with concomitant IV heparin reduced 30-day mortality by 14% relative to streptokinase (6.3% vs. 7.3%, p < 0.001).[87]

Table 5.1.   Management of ST-Elevation MI at Noninterventional Centers: Randomized Trials of On-site Lytic Therapy vs. Hospital Transfer for PCI

Trial	Design	Results (PCI vs. Lytic)	Comments
DANAMI-2 (2002)[47]	1129 patients with MI < 12 hours and ST-elevation ≥ 4 mm randomized to on-site accelerated tPA or transfer for PCI if transfer time < 3 hours	Death, reinfarction, or disabling stroke at 30 days* (8.5% vs. 14.2%, p = 0.0003); death at 30 days (6.6% vs. 7.6%, p = 0.35); stroke at 30 days (1.1% vs. 2.0%, p = 0.15)	Transport time ~ 60 minutes. Few complications during transport (VF 1.4%, high-degree AV block 2.3%). Door to-balloon time 100 minutes in transport group. Stents placed in 93%. Low rate (2.5%) of rescue PCI in tPA group
PRAGUE-2 (2002)[49a]	850 patients with MI < 12 hours randomized to streptokinase or immediate transport for PCI	Death at 30 days* (6.8% vs. 10%, p = 0.12); patients treated at 3-12 hours (6% vs. 15.3%, p < 0.02)	Death or VF during transport 1.2%. Transport increased time to treatment by 32 minutes
PRAGUE (2000)[49]	300 patients with ST-elevation MI < 6 hours randomized to lytic therapy in community hospital, lytic therapy during transport for PCI, or immediate transport for PCI	Death, reinfarction, or stroke at 30 days* (23% vs. 15% vs. 8%, p < 0.02); reinfarction at 30 days (10% vs. 7% vs. 1%, p < 0.03)	VF during transport: 2% with lytics during transport vs. 0% without lytics during transport

* Primary endpoint

Genetic recombinant technology has developed new fibrinolytic agents in the last few years, including rPA and TNK-tPA, which offer the convenience of IV bolus dosing and achieve similar patency rates as accelerated tPA. Numerous trials are underway evaluating various combinations of fibrinolytics, antithrombins, and GP IIb/IIIa inhibitors. Results of ASSENT-3 and GUSTO-V have recently been published (pp. 55-56).

B. Time-Dependent Benefits. Mortality rates are cut in half when fibrinolytic therapy is initiated within 1 hour of acute MI and decline thereafter. For every 1000 patients treated, 65 lives are saved when lytics are given within 1 hour of symptom onset, 26 lives are saved between 3-6 hours, and 18 lives are saved between 6-12 hours.[7] Patients with stuttering infarcts may benefit from fibrinolytic therapy for up to 24 hours. In a pooled analysis of 10 randomized trials of fibrinolytic therapy vs. primary angioplasty, the combined rate of death, reinfarction, and stroke at 30 days for patients presenting < 2 hours, 2-4 hours, and > 4 hours from symptom onset was 12.5%, 14.2%, and 19.6%, respectively.[43] Fibrinolytic therapy improves outcomes in all patient subsets, regardless of age, gender, blood pressure (if systolic BP < 180 mmHg), site of infarction, history of MI, or presence of diabetes or heart failure. Benefits are greatest for patients with new left bundle branch block or anterior ST-elevation; benefits are reduced in the very elderly due to an increased risk of major bleeding and in low-risk patients with small infarcts (e.g., inferior MI without RV infarction or anterior ST-depression), who have a good prognosis even without fibrinolytic therapy.

C. Limitations of Fibrinolytic Therapy. Important limitations of fibrinolytic therapy include acute patency rates ≤ 80%, failure to achieve optimal tissue reperfusion in 50%, intracranial hemorrhage in 0.5-1.5%, recurrent ischemia in 15-30%, and limited patient eligibility. Fibrinolytic therapy also activates platelets by exposing clot-bound thrombin.

Table 5.2. Fibrinolytic Therapy: Indications and Contraindications

Indications
- Patients with ST-segment elevation or LBBB who present within 12 hours of symptom onset, regardless of age, gender, site of infarction, presence of heart failure or diabetes, or history of MI
- Patients with isolated ST-segment depression with upright T waves and dominant R waves in leads V_1-V_2, consistent with posterior MI from left circumflex coronary occlusion

Contraindications
- Hemorrhagic stroke at any time in past
- Ischemic stroke or other cerebrovascular events within 1 year
- Known intracranial neoplasm
- Suspected aortic dissection
- Active internal bleeding (excluding menses)

Cautions/Relative Contraindications
- History of chronic severe hypertension
- Severe uncontrolled hypertension at presentation (BP > 180/110 mmHg)*
- Prior cerebrovascular accident or known intracerebral pathology not covered in contraindications
- Current use of anticoagulants in therapeutic doses (INR ≥ 2-3) or known bleeding diathesis
- Recent trauma (within 2-4 weeks), including head trauma or traumatic or prolonged (> 10 min) CPR or major surgery (within 3 weeks)
- Active peptic ulcer disease
- Recent (within 2-4 weeks) internal bleeding
- Noncompressible vascular punctures
- Pregnancy
- For streptokinase/anistreplase, prior exposure (especially within 5 days to 2 years) or prior allergic reaction

* Could be an absolute contraindication in low-risk patients.
Adapted from: ACC/AHA Guidelines for the Management of Patients with Acute Myocardial Infarction. J Am Coll Cardiol 1999;34:890-911.

Choice of Fibrinolytic Agent

No fibrinolytic agent is ideal for all patients, and each has its own advantages and disadvantages (Table 5.3). tPA, rPA, and TNK-tPA activate plasminogen directly, while streptokinase binds to plasminogen to form an "activator complex" (Figure 5.1).[86] Ultimately, plasminogen is converted to plasmin, which degrades fibrin clots. Fibrin-specific agents (tPA, TNK-tPA) preferentially activate clot-bound plasminogen, promoting clot lysis without inducing a systemic lytic state. In addition to activating clot-bound plasminogen, streptokinase, and to a lesser degree, rPA, activate *circulating* plasminogen, which degrades circulating fibrinogen and other plasma proteins to induce a systemic lytic state, manifest as elevated of fibrin degradation products, low fibrinogen levels, and depletion of clotting factors V and VIII. Compared to streptokinase, tPA resulted in higher acute patency rates (80% vs. 50%) and a 1% absolute reduction in early mortality (6.3% vs. 7.3%) in GUSTO-I,[87] but tPA requires IV heparin, results in more intracranial hemorrhage, and is more expensive. tPA, rPA, and TNK-tPA appear to be equivalent clinically, but there are differences in the ease of administration (TNK-tPA = single IV bolus; rPA = double IV bolus; tPA = IV bolus plus 90-minute infusion) and the risk of bleeding complications. Compared to tPA, TNK-tPA resulted in fewer major bleeding complications, fewer blood transfusions, less intracranial hemorrhage (ICH) in low-weight elderly women, and a trend toward less ICH in patients > 75 years in ASSENT-2.[88] Compared to tPA, rPA resulted in more bleeding complications in low-weight patients in GUSTO-III.[89,90] As of early 2003, TNK-tPA has the most convincing data for clinical benefit and ease of administration; rPA also has acceptable data, and streptokinase is preferred by some for patients at high risk of intracranial bleeding. Until ongoing trials are completed, either low-molecular-weight heparin (enoxaparin) or unfractionated heparin can be used as adjunctive antithrombin therapy.

Table 5.3. Fibrinolytic Agents for Acute MI

Agent	Dose	Comments
Streptokinase (SK)	1.5 million units (MU) IV over 30-60 minutes	Acute patency rate: 50%. Activates circulating plasminogen to induce a systemic lytic state. Allergic reactions are common (most often hypotension). Least likely to cause intracranial bleeding.[87,113,114] Acute IV heparin is not necessary for reduction in mortality or reinfarction,[87] and subcutaneous heparin is of questionable benefit.[113,114] Consider heparin in high-risk settings.[‡] Avoid reuse for ≥ 2 years due to the persistence of neutralizing anti-streptococcal antibodies. Least expensive lytic ($520*)
Tissue plasminogen activator (tPA) (Alteplase)	100 mg IV maximum in 90 minutes: 15 mg bolus, then 0.75 mg/kg (max. 50 mg) over 30 minutes, then 0.5 mg/kg (max. 35 mg) over next 60 minutes	Acute patency rate: 80%. Preferentially activates clot-bound plasminogen; does not induce a systemic lytic state. No allergic potential. Mortality advantage over SK if accelerated dosing regimen and IV heparin are given within 4 hours of symptom onset despite a slight increase in ICH.[87] Greatest benefit is for patients presenting early with large MI and low risk of ICH. Acute IV heparin[‡‡] is essential to maintain coronary patency. Expensive ($2600*)
Recombinant plasminogen activator (rPA) (Reteplase)	10 U IV bolus over 2 minutes, repeated in 30 minutes x 1. Normal saline flush before and after each bolus	Acute patency rate: 80%. Preferentially activates clot-bound plasminogen, but not as fibrin-specific as tPA, and fibrinogen is depleted in many patients. No allergic potential. Deletion mutant of wild-type tPA with a longer half-life and reduced fibrin specificity compared to tPA. Convenient bolus dosing. Mortality and ICH similar to accelerated tPA in GUSTO-III.[89,115] Acute IV heparin[‡‡] is essential to maintain coronary patency. Expensive ($2650*)

See footnotes, next page.

Table 5.3. Fibrinolytic Agents for Acute MI (cont'd)

Agent	Dose	Comments
TNK-tPA (Tenecteplase)	Single, weight-adjusted IV bolus over 5 seconds: < 60 kg (30 mg); 60-69 kg (35 mg); 70-79 kg (40 mg); 80-89 kg (45 mg); ≥ 90 kg (50 mg)	Acute patency rate: 80%. Preferentially activates clot-bound plasminogen; does not induce a systemic lytic state. No allergic potential. Developed by altering amino acids of wild-type tPA; longer half-life and increased fibrin specificity compared to tPA. Convenient bolus dosing. Mortality and ICH similar to accelerated tPA in ASSENT-2.[88] Acute IV heparin[‡‡] is essential to maintain coronary patency. Expensive ($2650*)

ICH = intracranial hemorrhage

* Pharmacy cost at Duke Hospital

‡ Consider IV infusion of unfractionated heparin at 12-15 U/kg/hr for patients at high risk of thromboembolism (e.g., large anterior MI, previous embolus, atrial fibrillation, LV thrombus). Begin after 4-6 hours or when aPTT < 2-3 times control and continue for 2-5 days. Titrate to aPTT of 1.5-2.5 times control (50-75 seconds). Alternatively, subcutaneous heparin can be given at 12,500 U q12h, starting at 4-12 hours and continued for 3-7 days. Patients at low risk of thromboembolism can be treated either without heparin or with low-dose (7500 U) subcutaneous heparin q12h until ambulatory.

‡‡ Unfractionated heparin IV bolus of 60-70 U/kg (max. 5000 units) followed by an IV infusion of 12-15 U/kg/hr (max. 1000 U/hr), adjusted to aPTT of 1.5-2.5 times control (50-75 seconds) x 48 hours. Alternatively, enoxaparin can be administered at 1 mg/kg (SQ) q12h (consider initial bolus dose of 30 mg IV as in ASSENT-3 trial).

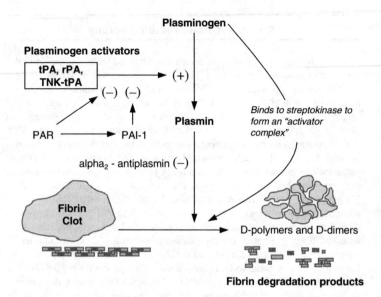

Figure 5.1. Fibrinolytic Therapy and Dissolution of Clot

Fibrinolytic agents activate plasminogen, which degrades thrombus via breakdown of fibrin. tPA, rPA, and TNK-tPA activate plasminogen directly; streptokinase combines with plasminogen to form an "activator complex." Fibrin breakdown results in the release of fibrin degradation products (D-dimers and other D-polymers). PAI = plasminogen activator inhibitor.

Adjunctive Antithrombin Therapy

Fibrinolytic therapy exposes clot-bound thrombin, which is a potent stimulus for further platelet aggregation and fibrin generation.[86] To offset this prothrombotic potential, antithrombin therapy is routinely employed, particularly with tPA, rPA, and TNK-tPA. There is less need for systemic anticoagulation with streptokinase, as streptokinase results in the generation of fibrin degradation products and the depletion of clotting factors V and VIII, which confer systemic anticoagulant effects. Heparin dosing is a balance between the risk of reocclusion and the risk of major bleeding, and current guidelines recommend an IV bolus dose of 60-70 U/kg (max. 5000 units) of unfractionated heparin (UFH) followed by a continuous IV infusion of 12-15 U/kg/hr (max. 1000 U/hr), adjusted to aPTT of 1.5-2.5 times control (50-75 seconds) x 48 hours (Table 5.4).[91,92] As alternatives to UFH, bivalirudin (direct thrombin inhibitor) and enoxaparin (low-molecular-weight heparin) have recently been evaluated during fibrinolytic therapy. As an adjunct to streptokinase in HERO-2, bivalirudin reduced the rate of reinfarction at 96 hours by 30% compared to UFH but did not reduce mortality at 30 days.[93] As an adjunct to TNK-tPA in ASSENT-3, enoxaparin reduced the primary endpoint of 30-day mortality or hospital reinfarction or refractory ischemia by 19% compared to UFH (11.4% vs. 15.4%, p = 0.0001, p. 55).[94] Given enoxaparin's ease of administration, lack of need for monitoring, and potential clinical benefit over UFH, results of ongoing trials with enoxaparin in ST-elevation MI are eagerly awaited.

Management of Lytic Complications

A. **Minor Bleeding (puncture site, oral, nasal).** Minor bleeding episodes are treated by local compression. To minimize the risk of bleeding, compressible vascular access sites should be used, vascular access lines should be left in place for several hours after fibrinolytic therapy (especially after streptokinase), and the number of invasive procedures should be kept to a minimum.

B. **Major Bleeding (GI, intracranial).** The incidence of GI bleeding is 5% and intracranial hemorrhage is 0.5-1.0% after fibrinolytic therapy. Risk

Table 5.4. Heparin Dosage Adjustment With Fibrinolytic Therapy for Acute MI*

aPTT (sec)	Bolus Dose (units)	Stop Infusion (min)	Rate Changes (mL/hr)	Repeat aPTT
< 40	3000	0	+2	6 hours
40-49	0	0	+1	6 hours
50-75	0	0	0 (no changes)	Next AM
76-85	0	0	−1	Next AM
86-100	0	30	−2	6 hours
101-150	0	60	−3	6 hours
>150	0	60	−6	6 hours

aPTT = activated partial thromboplastin time. Heparin infusion concentration = 50 U/mL. Target aPTT = 50-75 seconds.

* For standard laboratory reagents with a mean control aPTT of 26-36 seconds. For aPTT obtained < 6 hours after fibrinolytic therapy, adjust infusion upward if aPTT < 50 seconds, but only down-titrate for aPTT > 100 seconds as the aPTT will be affected by the lytic state. For aPTT obtained ≥ 12 hours after fibrinolytic therapy, use nomogram as above. Modified from: Chest 1995;108:258S-275S.

factors for intracranial hemorrhage, which is fatal in 50-60%, include older age (especially > 70 years), lower body weight, history of cerebrovascular events, hypertension on presentation, and use of a fibrin-specific fibrinolytic agent. Any focal neurological deficit or significant deterioration in mental status should be treated as an intracranial hemorrhage until excluded by CT scan. STAT blood counts (hemoglobin, hematocrit, platelets, PT/PTT, fibrinogen) should be obtained and treatment should be started before CT results are available. Immediate discontinuation of lytics, heparin, GP IIb/IIIa inhibitors, aspirin, and clopidogrel is mandatory. Protamine sulfate (20-50 mg IV over 1-3 minutes) can be given to reverse the effects of heparin. Packed RBCs are indicated for bleeding-induced hypotension or hematocrit < 25%; platelet transfusions (6-10 units) are indicated to reverse abciximab effects; and cryoprecipitate (10 units IV) is indicated to keep fibrinogen levels > 150 mg/dL. (Fibrinogen can be low or dysfunctional 6-8 hours after tPA, rPA, and TNK-tPA, and for up to 30 hours after streptokinase.) For persistent bleeding, fresh frozen plasma (2-3 units IV) and repeat cryoprecipitate transfusions are indicated. For continued bleeding despite these measures, additional platelet transfusions (even if the platelet count is normal) are recommended to reverse the effect of aspirin and fibrin split products. Aminocaproic acid may counteract the effect of plasmin but at a risk of severe thrombosis.

C. **Fever.** Fever occurs in 5% of patients receiving streptokinase and is treated with aspirin or acetaminophen.

D. **Hypotension.** Hypotension occurs in 10-15% of patients during streptokinase infusions and is treated with IV fluids and by slowing or temporarily discontinuing the streptokinase infusion until BP > 90 mmHg, then resuming the normal infusion rate. Hypotension is not an allergic reaction unless it is associated with anaphylaxis.

E. **Rash.** Rash occurs in 2-3% of patients receiving streptokinase and is treated by discontinuing the streptokinase infusion and giving benadryl 50 mg (IV or PO) and hydrocortisone 100 mg (IV) q6h (if severe). If a full lytic dose was not received, 50 mg tPA or acute PCI should be considered.

F. **Anaphylaxis.** Anaphylaxis occurs in 0.1% of patients receiving streptokinase and is treated by discontinuing the streptokinase infusion, securing an airway, and giving epinephrine 1-5 cc of 1:10,000 solution IV, hydrocortisone 100-200 mg IV q4-6h x 24h, and IV fluids. IV dopamine 5-20 mcg/kg/min or norepinephrine 0.5-30 mcg/min is indicated for persistent hypotension, and albuterol 0.5 cc of 0.5% solution in 2-5 cc normal saline as an aerosolized mist is useful for bronchospasm.

G. **Rigors.** Rigors can occur during plasminogen breakdown and are treated with demerol 25 mg IV.

H. **Reperfusion Arrhythmias**
   1. **Bradycardia, 3° AV block.** Occurs most often with acute reperfusion of the right coronary artery (RCA) and usually resolves within minutes. Symptomatic episodes are treated with atropine 0.5-1.0 mg IV every 3-5 minutes and IV fluids. Transcutaneous pacing is rarely needed.
   2. **Bezold-Jarish reflex.** Presents as profound hypotension with bradycardia in response to activation of vagal afferent fibers following acute reperfusion of the RCA. Treated with atropine 0.5-1.0 mg IV every 3-5 minutes, IV fluids, and possibly temporary pacing. Persistent episodes may require norepinephrine 0.5-30 mcg/min IV.
   3. **Idioventricular rhythm.** No treatment is required for rates < 120 bpm in the absence of hypotension.

4. **Ventricular tachycardia (VT).** No treatment is required for runs of nonsustained VT, which are common and usually abate over time. For pulseless VT or ventricular fibrillation, immediate defibrillation is required (p. 115).

PCI After Fibrinolytic Therapy

Several interventional approaches are available for the management of acute MI after lytic therapy, including rescue, immediate, and delayed PCI (Table 5.5). Most randomized trials evaluating these approaches were conducted prior to the widespread availability of stents and GP IIb/IIIa inhibitors, which have greatly improved the safety and efficacy of PCI.

A. **Rescue (Salvage) PCI for Failed Fibrinolysis.** In small randomized trials of PTCA vs. medical therapy for failed lytic therapy, successful PTCA improved regional and global LV function, and there was a trend toward less recurrent ischemia, heart failure, shock, and death in high-risk patients.[95-99] However, early mortality was high (30-40%) when rescue PTCA was unsuccessful.[100,101] Stenting appears to improve the results of rescue PCI. In 83 patients who underwent rescue stenting, TIMI-3 flow was achieved in 93%, and there were low rates of major adverse cardiac events (death, reinfarction, CABG, or target lesion revascularization) during hospitalization (3.6%) and at 1 year (18.8%), similar to results obtained with primary stenting for acute MI.[102] In the GUSTO-III substudy (nonrandomized), there was a trend toward lower 30-day mortality when abciximab was used during rescue angioplasty (3.6% vs. 9.7%, p = 0.076).[98] Emergency angiography should be considered for patients with ongoing chest pain, hemodynamic instability, or persistent ST-elevation 90 minutes after lytic therapy for anterior MI. Stenting with GP IIb/IIIa inhibitors is recommended for high-grade lesions with TIMI flow ≤ 2.

B. **Immediate PCI After Successful Fibrinolysis in Asymptomatic Patients.** Immediate PTCA for significant residual stenosis in asymptomatic patients resulted in higher rates of blood transfusion, emergency CABG, and death compared to no intervention,[103-105] but these studies were limited by inconsistent use of preprocedural aspirin and ACT monitoring. Contemporary small studies (PACT) suggest that angioplasty can be performed safely immediately following fibrinolytic therapy.[67] The ASSENT IV trial is testing this strategy in the current era.

Table 5.5. PCI Approaches After Fibrinolytic Therapy for Acute MI

Approach	Description
Rescue (salvage) PCI	PCI after failed fibrinolysis (TIMI 0-1 blood flow in the infarct vessel)
Immediate PCI	PCI for significant residual stenosis immediately after successful fibrinolysis
Delayed (deferred) PCI	PCI for significant residual stenosis 1-7 days after fibrinolysis (prior to discharge)

PCI = percutaneous coronary intervention

C. **Delayed (1-7 days) PCI After Successful Fibrinolysis in Asymptomatic Patients.** Randomized trials (TIMI-2B,[106] SWIFT[107]) comparing invasive (routine PTCA before discharge) and conservative (PTCA for spontaneous or inducible ischemia) approaches following successful fibrinolysis showed no difference in death, reinfarction, or LV ejection fraction. However, in TIMI-2B, intraprocedural ACT was not monitored, total occlusions were not dilated, and intention-to-treat analysis may have attenuated the beneficial effect of PTCA, since only 54% of patients in the invasive arm received PTCA and the majority of deaths in the invasive arm occurred prior to revascularization. It is reasonable to consider predischarge angiography in patients with LV dysfunction, known multivessel disease, or prior MI/CABG, followed by stenting with a GP IIb/IIIa inhibitor for high-grade stenoses supplying moderate or large areas of viable myocardium.

D. **Delayed PCI of an Occluded Vessel After Failed Fibrinolysis in Asymptomatic Patients.** TAMI-6 reported improved ejection fraction at 6 weeks in patients treated with PTCA at 48 hours compared to those treated medically, but 40% of vessels were reoccluded at 6 months.[108] Nonrandomized studies reported better survival after successful PTCA,[109-111] possibly due to improved ventricular remodeling, better recovery of viable but hibernating myocardium, and fewer arrhythmias. Data are limited, but late PCI of occluded infarct vessels should be considered if there is a large area of myocardium or evidence of viability (e.g., preserved wall motion, retained R-waves, PET viability, collaterals) in the territory of the infarct vessel. This strategy is being tested in the NIH-funded Open Artery Trial

(OAT).

E. PCI for Recurrent Ischemia After Fibrinolysis. Compared to a strategy of PTCA for refractory symptoms only, PTCA for spontaneous or inducible ischemia after fibrinolytic therapy reduced the incidence of MI, unstable angina, and use of anti-ischemic drugs in DANAMI, and there was a trend towards a reduction in death long term..[112] Patients with post-infarct angina or an abnormal stress test should undergo cardiac catheterization and revascularization based on anatomy.

New Reperfusion Strategies for Acute MI

Fibrinolytic therapy exposes clot-bound thrombin, which is a potent platelet activator, and TIMI-3 flow rates are achieved in only 50-60% of infarct vessels after fibrinolytic therapy. Furthermore, microvascular embolization of platelet aggregates may impair myocardial reperfusion despite good epicardial blood flow.[116] To offset the prothrombotic potential of fibrinolytic therapy, recent trials have evaluated the role for GP IIb/IIIa inhibitors and/or enoxaparin as adjuncts to fibrinolytic therapy.

A. Full-Dose Fibrinolysis Plus GP IIb/IIIa Inhibitor. TAMI 8 evaluated the safety of tPA (100 mg), aspirin, and graded-doses of abciximab in patients with acute MI and demonstrated a dose-dependent reduction in platelet aggregation with increasing doses of abciximab.[117] In IMPACT-AMI, the addition of eptifibatide to tPA increased the speed and frequency of reperfusion, without an increase in bleeding.[118] In PARADIGM,[119] there was no improvement in clinical outcome and more bleeding complications with the addition of lamifiban to tPA or streptokinase, but ST-segment monitoring indicated that lamifiban resulted in more rapid reperfusion.

B. Low-Dose Fibrinolysis Plus GP IIb/IIIa Inhibitor. The TIMI 14a Pilot study found that half-dose tPA combined with standard-dose abciximab resulted in TIMI-3 flow in 79% at 90 minutes.[120] In SPEED, half-dose rPA plus standard-dose abciximab resulted in TIMI-3 flow in 73% at 90 minutes.[121] Recently, results of the large, randomized, multicenter ASSENT-3[122] and GUSTO-V[123] trials have been published.

    1. ASSENT-3 (Table 5.6). In this trial, 6095 patients with acute MI < 6 hours and ST-elevation or LBBB were randomized to one of three drug regimens: (1) full-dose TNK-tPA plus unfractionated heparin (UFH); (2) half-dose TNK-tPA plus abciximab plus UFH; (3) full-dose TNK-tPA plus enoxaparin. Compared to TNK-tPA plus UFH, the primary efficacy endpoint (30-day mortality or in-hospital reinfarction or refractory ischemia) was reduced in the enoxaparin and abciximab groups. The composite endpoint of primary efficacy, in-hospital intracranial hemorrhage, and major bleeding complications was reduced with enoxaparin but not with abciximab. Abciximab was associated with worse outcome in elderly patients (age > 75 years), no benefit in diabetics, and increased bleeding complications in diabetics and the elderly.[122]

    2. **GUSTO-V (Table 5.7).** In this trial, 16,588 patients with acute MI < 6 hours and ST-elevation or LBBB were treated with UFH and randomized to full-dose rPA or half-dose rPA plus abciximab. There was no difference in 30-day mortality (primary endpoint), but half-dose rPA plus abciximab resulted in less death or reinfarction at 30 days (7.4% vs. 8.8%, p = 0.0011), less need for urgent PCI, less reinfarction or recurrent ischemia at 7 days, but more major bleeding complications (1.1% vs. 0.5%, p < 0.0001). Patients over age 75 had a higher rate of intracranial hemorrhage with half-dose rPA plus abciximab (2.1% vs. 1.1%), but those under age 75 had a lower rate of intracranial hemorrhage (0.4% vs. 0.5%). At 1 year, mortality rates were identical between groups (8.4%), although there was a trend towards lower mortality in patients < 75 years with anterior MI who received half-dose rPA plus abciximab (7.1% vs. 8.0%, p = 0.21).[123]

C. **Full-Dose Fibrinolysis Plus Low-Molecular-Weight Heparin (LMWH).** LMWH has several advantages over unfractionated heparin (UFH) (p. 87), and enoxaparin was associated with less death or MI compared to UFH in randomized trials of non-ST-elevation ACS (p. 90). Compared to UFH in ASSENT-3, the addition of enoxaparin to TNK-tPA for ST-elevation MI reduced the primary composite endpoint (30-day death or in-hospital reinfarction or refractory ischemia) by 26% (11.4% vs. 15.4%, p = 0.0001), with only a modest increase in major bleeding but with need for additional data, especially in the elderly (Table 5.6).[122] The ENTIRE trial is evaluating enoxaparin vs. UFH in 25,000 patients treated with the 4 most commonly used lytics.

D. Recommendations. Reperfusion strategies combining standard- or low-dose fibrinolytic therapy with a GP IIb/IIIa inhibitor, enoxaparin, or a direct thrombin inhibitor may enhance reperfusion and reduce ischemic complications in ST-elevation MI. Ongoing trials will help determine the optimal combination, dose, and timing for these various approaches.

Table 5.6. Results of the ASSENT-3 Trial[122]

Outcomes	Full-dose TNK-tPA[1] + enoxaparin[2] (n = 2040)	Half-dose TNK-tPA + abciximab[3] + UFH[4] (n = 2017)	Full-dose TNK-tPA[1] + UFH[5] (n = 2038)	p-Value
30-day death or in-hospital reinfarction or refractory ischemia (primary endpoint) (%)	11.4	11.1	15.4	0.0001
Primary endpoint or in-hospital ICH or major bleeding (%)	13.8	14.2	17.0	0.0081
Death at 30 days (%)	5.4	6.6	6.0	0.25
In-hospital events (%)				
Reinfarction	2.7	2.2	4.2	0.0009
Refractory ischemia	4.6	3.2	6.5	< 0.0001
ICH	0.9	0.9	0.9	0.98
Major bleeding (non-ICH)	3.0	4.3	2.2	0.0005

ICH = intracranial hemorrhage, MI = myocardial infarction, TNK-tPA = tenecteplase, UFH = unfractionated heparin

1. TNK-tPA (single weight-adjusted IV bolus): 30 mg (< 60 kg); 35 mg (60-69 kg); 40 mg (70-79 kg); 45 mg (80-89 kg); 50 mg (≥ 90 kg)
2. Enoxaparin: 30 mg IV bolus followed immediately by 1 mg/kg SQ q12h up to 7 days (max. 100 mg SQ for first 2 doses)
3. Abciximab: 0.25 mg/kg IV bolus plus 0.125 mcg/kg/min IV infusion (max. 10 mcg/min) x 12 hours
4. Heparin with abciximab: 40 U/kg IV bolus (max. 3000 U) + 7 U/kg/hr IV infusion (max. 800 U/hr) to maintain aPTT at 50-70 seconds
5. Heparin without abciximab: 60 U/kg IV bolus (max. 4000 U) plus 12 U/kg/hr IV infusion (max. 1000 U/hr) to maintain aPTT at 50-70 seconds x 48 hours

From: Lancet 2001;357;1905-14

Table 5.7. Results of the GUSTO-V Trial[123]

Outcomes	rPA[1] (n = 8260)	Half-dose rPA + abciximab[2] (n = 8328)	p-Value
30-days (%)			
Death (primary endpoint)	5.9	5.6	0.43
Death or nonfatal MI	8.8	7.4	0.0011
Up to day 7 (%)			
Reinfarction	3.5	2.3	< 0.0001
Recurrent ischemia	12.8	11.3	0.004
Urgent PCI < 6 hrs	8.6	5.6	< 0.0001
Severe bleeding	0.5	1.1	< 0.0001
Transfusion	4.0	5.7	< 0.0001
ICH			
> 75 years	1.1	2.1	< 0.02*
≤ 75 years	0.5	0.4	
1-year mortality (%)			
All patients	8.4	8.4	NS
Age < 75 years with anterior MI	8.0	7.1	0.21

ICH = intracranial hemorrhage, MI = myocardial infarction, PCI = percutaneous coronary intervention, rPA = reteplase

* For interaction by age

1. rPA: 10 U bolus x 2, 30 minutes apart. Heparin: 5000 U IV bolus plus an IV infusion of 1000 U/hr (> 80 kg) or 800 U/hr (< 80 kg) to maintain aPTT at 50-70 seconds
2. rPA: 5 U IV bolus x 2, 30 minutes apart. Abciximab: 0.25 mg/kg IV bolus plus 0.125 mcg/kg/min IV infusion (max. 10 mcg/min) x 12 hours. Heparin: 60 U/kg IV bolus (max. 5000 U) + 7 U/kg/hr IV infusion

From: Lancet 2001:358:605-13. One-year mortality results presented at XIVth World Congress of Cardiology, Sydney, Australia, 2002.

Section 3

NON-ST-ELEVATION ACS

Chapter 6. Diagnosis and Evaluation 58
Chapter 7. Overview of Management 63
Chapter 8. Interventional Management 70
Chapter 9. Drug Therapy 75
Chapter 10. Special Patient Populations 94

Chapter 6

Diagnosis and Evaluation of
Non-ST-Elevation ACS

Patients with non-ST-elevation ACS cannot be divided into categories of
unstable angina or acute MI until serum biomarkers of myocardial necrosis
become available. These patients are initially grouped together, since their
pathophysiology, presentation, and management are similar.

Diagnosis

A. **Unstable Angina.** Unstable angina is a clinical diagnosis. Based on the
   onset, duration, and frequency of chest pain, unstable angina can be
   categorized into rest angina, new-onset severe angina, or increasing
   angina.[124] ECG changes may or may not be present, and serum cardiac
   markers are normal.
   1. **Rest angina.** Angina that occurs at rest, usually within a week of
      presentation. Episodes are often prolonged (> 20 minutes).
   2. **New-onset severe angina.** New onset of class III-IV angina. Angina
      occurs after walking ≤ 1-2 blocks on a flat surface or climbing ≤ 1 flight
      of stairs at normal pace.
   3. **Increasing angina**. Previously diagnosed angina that is distinctly more
      frequent, longer, or lower in threshold. There is at least 1 functional
      class increase to class III or IV severity.

B. **Non-ST-Elevation MI.** The diagnosis of acute MI requires one of two
   criteria. The first criterion requires the rise and fall of cardiac markers
   (troponin or CK-MB) *plus* one of the following: symptoms of ischemia, Q
   waves or ischemic changes on ECG, or coronary intervention. The second
   criterion is pathological findings indicative of acute MI.[1] There are
   important limitations to these criteria: acute MI can present with atypical
   symptoms, noncardiac disorders can manifest ischemic-type chest pain and
   ST-segment changes, and the rise and fall in cardiac markers is time-
   dependent and can be missed.

Symptoms

The most common presentation for non-ST-elevation ACS is chest, neck, or jaw discomfort, which is usually described as pressure, burning, or squeezing in character. Symptoms typically last < 30 minutes in unstable angina and > 30 minutes in non-ST-elevation MI. Atypical presentations—weakness, dyspnea, heart failure—are more common in diabetics and the elderly, and women may present with dyspnea or jaw pain stretched out over hours, rather than minutes. Pleuritic-type symptoms and pain reproduced by palpation are very unusual presentations but do not exclude the possibility of ACS. Up to 20% of infarcts are "silent" or go unrecognized by the physician or patient. Silent MI occurs most often in diabetics with autonomic dysfunction.

Electrocardiogram

Patients with non-ST-elevation ACS can present with ischemic ST-segment and T-wave changes, nonspecific ST-T changes, or a relatively normal ECG.[125] An interesting group will have transient ST-segment elevation followed by one of the aforementioned patterns. ECG changes can be persistent, evident only during chest pain, or they may not occur at all. Classic ischemic changes include horizontal or downsloping ST-depression ≥ 0.5 mm and/or symmetrically inverted T-waves > 2.0 (Figure 6.1). Deep T-wave inversions across the precordial leads strongly suggest severe stenosis of the left anterior descending (LAD) coronary artery.[126] Ischemic T-waves can also be biphasic or upright and peaked (hyperacute). Patients with dynamic ST-T changes are at increased risk of death or MI [2,127] and are managed more aggressively than patients without ECG changes or other high-risk markers.[128] It is important to obtain serial ECGs in patients with ongoing chest pain and normal or nonspecific changes on initial ECG, since some patients develop complete coronary occlusion and ST-elevation during hospitalization and benefit from reperfusion therapy. Continuous ECG monitoring with attention to ST-segment shifts can be used for this purpose. "Ischemic" ECG changes lack specificity for coronary artery disease and can be seen in a variety of non-ischemic conditions (Table 6.1).

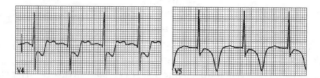

Figure 6.1. ST and T-Wave Changes in Non-ST-Elevation ACS

Table 6.1. Differential Diagnosis for "Ischemic" ECG Changes[6]

ST-Segment Depression	Deeply Inverted T-Waves	Tall Peaked T-Waves
• Myocardial ischemia • Repolarization changes secondary to ventricular hypertrophy or IVCD • Digitalis effect • "Pseudodepression" from superimposition of atrial flutter waves or prominent atrial repolarization wave on the ST segment, as seen in atrial enlargement, pericarditis, or atrial infarction • CNS disorder • Hypokalemia • Quinidine effect • Mitral valve prolapse	• Myocardial ischemia • LVH • RVH • CNS disorder • WPW Syndrome	• Acute MI (hyperacute T-waves) • Angina pectoris • Normal variant (usually mid-precordial leads) • Hyperkalemia (more common when acute) • Intracranial bleeding • LVH • RVH • LBBB • Pseudo-peaked T waves from superimposition of P waves on the T wave, as seen with APCs, sinus rhythm with marked 1° AV block, or complete heart block • Anemia

APC = atrial premature contraction, AV = atrio-ventricular, CNS = central nervous system, IVCD = intraventricular conduction delay, LBBB = left bundle branch block, LVH = left ventricular hypertrophy, MI = myocardial infarction, RVH = right ventricular hypertrophy, WPW = Wolff-Parkinson-White

Serum Cardiac Markers

CK-MB and cardiac troponin levels are used to differentiate unstable angina from acute MI, assess prognosis, and guide therapy.[129] Cardiac markers should be obtained on admission and repeated at least once (troponin) or twice (CK-MB) at 6-8 hour intervals. Elevated cardiac troponin levels are associated with 3-8–fold increased risk of death or MI and identify patients most likely to benefit from GP IIb/IIIa inhibitors and the invasive approach to management.[15-22] No single cardiac marker is ideal, and each has its own advantages and disadvantages (pp. 16-17). Since cardiac markers may not turn positive for hours, early treatment is based on clinical presentation and the initial ECG. Elevated levels of acute phase reactants (C-reactive protein, interleukin-6, amyloid A) also predict adverse outcome.

Other Studies

Hemoglobin, platelet count, serum lipids, and other routine serum chemistries should be obtained in the emergency department. A chest x-ray is recommended on admission in hemodynamically-unstable patients and within 48 hours in stable patients.

Risk Stratification

All patients with non-ST-elevation ACS should be classified according to their risk of short-term death or nonfatal MI (Table 6.2). In addition to providing prognostic information, risk categories serve as the basis for initial management decisions, which range from immediate angiography, GP IIb/IIIa inhibitors, and PCI (if indicated) for high-risk patients to outpatient management similar to chronic stable angina for low-risk patients.

Table 6.2. Short-Term Risk of Death or MI in Unstable Angina[128]

High Risk	Intermediate Risk	Low Risk
At least one feature must be present: • Prolonged (> 20 min) ongoing rest pain • Angina at rest with dynamic ST-depression ≥ 0.5 mm or new bundle branch block • Angina with new or worsening MR murmur • Angina with S_3, new or worsening rales, or pulmonary edema • Angina with hypotension, bradycardia, or tachycardia • Age ≥ 75 years • Elevated cardiac troponins (> 0.1 ng/mL) • Sustained ventricular tachycardia	No high-risk features but must have one of the following: • Prolonged (> 20 min) rest angina, now resolved, with moderate or high likelihood of coronary heart disease • Rest angina (< 20 min) relieved with rest or sublingual nitroglycerin • Angina with dynamic T-wave changes > 2.0 mm or abnormal Q-waves • Aspirin use • Prior MI or CABG • Peripheral vascular disease or cerebrovascular disease • Slightly elevated cardiac troponins (> 0.01 ng/mL but < 0.1 ng/mL) • Age > 70 years	No high- or-intermediate-risk features but may have any of the following: • New-onset angina or progressive CCS class III-IV angina without prolonged (> 20 min) chest pain but with moderate or high likelihood of coronary heart disease • Normal or unchanged ECG during chest discomfort • Cardiac markers not elevated

CCS = Canadian Cardiovascular Society, MR = mitral regurgitation. Adapted from: ACC/AHA Guideline Update for the Management of Patients with Unstable Angina or Non-ST-Elevation Myocardial Infarction, March, 2002

Chapter 7

Overview of Management of Non-ST-Elevation ACS (Figure 7.1)

Emergency Department Measures

All patients with non-ST-elevation ACS should be triaged to an invasive or conservative revascularization strategy based on risk category (Table 7.1). Hospitalized patients should receive aspirin (162-325 mg chewed followed by 75-325 mg PO q24h), beta-blockers (IV for ongoing pain; otherwise PO), and antithrombin therapy (enoxaparin or unfractionated heparin). Clopidogrel and GP IIb/IIIa inhibitor each provide benefit and their use is described on pp. 76-78. Clopidogrel should be withheld 5-7 days prior to CABG. Additional measures include nitroglycerin (sublingual tablet or spray) for ongoing pain, and morphine sulfate for pulmonary congestion, severe agitation, or ongoing pain despite nitrates. Verapamil, amlodipine, or diltiazem should be considered for ongoing or recurrent ischemia if beta-blockers are contraindicated and LV function is intact and for ACS due to variant angina or cocaine use. Nitrates should be avoided in RV infarction and within 24 hours of sildenafil (Viagra) (increased risk of severe hypotension),[133] immediate-release nifedipine should be avoided without a beta-blocker (increased risk of MI, recurrent angina, and death),[134] and fibrinolytics should be avoided due to their lack of clinical benefit and possible detrimental effect.[135] Other early measures include bed rest, peripheral access of a compressible vein, supplemental oxygen for respiratory distress or suspected hypoxemia, and control of precipitating factors (e.g., anemia, hypoxemia, hypovolemia, hypertension, hyperthyroidism, infection). Patients with refractory ischemia or hemodynamic instability despite medical therapy should be considered for intra-aortic balloon pump counterpulsation as a bridge to urgent PCI. Initial assessment should also exclude the presence of a life-threatening mimic of ACS: pulmonary embolism, aortic dissection, acute pericarditis, pneumothorax, esophageal rupture, or ischemia/rupture of an intra-abdominal organ.

Non-ST-Elevation ACS
(Unstable Angina or Non-ST-Elevation MI)

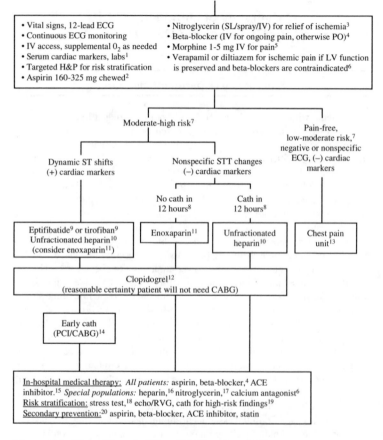

Figure 7.1. Management of Non-ST-Elevation ACS

See footnotes, next page.

Footnotes for Figure 7.1.

1. CK-MB every 6-8 hours x 3, cardiac troponins repeated at least once at 4-8 hours, complete blood count, platelet count, fibrinogen, lipid profile, electrolytes, BUN/creatinine, portable chest x-ray.
2. Buccal absorption of crushed or chewed nonenteric-coated aspirin produces the most rapid antiplatelet effects. Avoid enteric-coated preparations acutely due to delays in GI absorption and platelet inhibition. An aspirin suppository (325 mg) can be given to patients unable to take oral medications.
3. Up to 3 nitroglycerin tablets (0.4 mg) or 3 metered doses of nitroglycerin spray (0.4 mg) onto/under tongue at 5-minute intervals. Avoid if systolic BP < 90 mmHg, heart rate < 50 bpm, suspected RV infarction, or sildenafil (Viagra) use within 24 hours.
4. Avoid beta-blocker acutely if systolic BP < 90 mmHg, heart rate < 50 bpm, severe heart failure, or history of significant bronchospasm. Given IV followed by PO to patients with ongoing pain or high-risk features. Can start PO in low-risk asymptomatic patients. See p. 151 for dosing and administration guidelines.
5. Morphine can be repeated in small increments. Avoid in severe chronic lung disease (increased risk of respiratory depression). Hypoventilation can be reversed with naloxone (0.4-2.0 mg IV). Hypotension usually responds to leg elevation ± IV saline (200-300 cc if no pulmonary congestion). Bradycardia, nausea, and vomiting often improve with atropine (0.5-1.0 mg IV).
6. Diltiazem 120-320 mg/d (PO) or verapamil 120-480 mg/d (PO) in single or divided doses depending on the preparation. Also consider for non-Q-wave MI without pulmonary congestion, started on day 2-5 and continued up to 1 year.
7. See Table 6.2 (p. 62) for description of risk categories.
8. Early cath should be especially considered for patients with ongoing/recurrent pain, heart failure, hemodynamic instability, mitral regurgitation, or LV dysfunction. SYNERGY will determine if enoxaparin is preferred for cath < 12 hrs of presentation.
9. See Table 9.3 (p. 83) for dosing/administration guidelines for eptifibatide and tirofiban.
10. As medical therapy in conjunction with a GP IIb/IIIa inhibitor, UFH is given as 60-70 U/kg IV bolus (max. 5000 U) plus 12-15 U/kg/min (max. 1000 U/hr), adjusted to maintain aPTT at 1.5-2.5 times control (50-75 seconds).
11. Enoxaparin dose as primary medical therapy: 1 mg/kg SQ q12h x 2-8 days (optimal duration unknown). Enoxaparin dose as adjunct to PCI: 0.75 mg/kg IV if a GP IIb/IIIa inhibitor is to be used; 1 mg/kg IV if *no* GP IIb/IIIa inhibitor is planned. For patients treated with SQ enoxaparin and the last SQ dose is within 8 hours, no additional enoxaparin is required; if the last SQ dose is > 8 hours, an additional 0.3 mg/kg IV should be given just before PCI.
12. See discussion of clopidogrel for non-ST-elevation ACS (pp. 76-78).
13. For select patients with nondiagnostic or normal ECGs in whom the diagnosis of ACS is in doubt, one approach is to follow these patients in the emergency department for 8-12 hours and consider discharge to home if repeat serum cardiac markers are negative, serial ECGs remain stable, 2D echo (or possibly stress test) is normal, and

Footnotes for Figure 7.1 (cont'd)

there is no further evidence of ischemia. A stress test should be obtained within 48-72 hours if not performed in the emergency department prior to discharge.

14. Stent plus abciximab or eptifibatide (see Table 9.3, p. 83, for dosing regimens and use of adjunctive heparin/enoxaparin). Consider triage to CABG instead of PCI for significant left main disease, 3-vessel disease with treated diabetes or LV dysfunction, or 2-vessel disease with proximal LAD involvement and either LV dysfunction or ischemia on stress testing. Prior to CABG, discontinue clopidogrel x 5-7 days and GP IIb/IIIa inhibitors x several hours, and switch from enoxaparin to unfractionated heparin.

15. Start oral ACE inhibitor at low dose as soon as patient is stabilized from MI (after reperfusion and once blood pressure has stabilized; usually no sooner than 6 hours). Titrate upward over 1-4 days, as tolerated. See p. 148 for dosing and administration guidelines. Continue indefinitely if ejection fraction is reduced. For uncomplicated MI without LV dysfunction, discontinue after 4-6 weeks or consider long-term therapy for secondary prevention.

16. Consider continuing IV heparin (aPTT 50-75 seconds) for several days if the risk of thromboembolism is high (i.e., large anterior MI, LV thrombus, atrial fibrillation, prior embolism). Subcutaneous heparin 5000-7000 U q12h or enoxaparin 1 mg/kg q12h should be considered for others during periods of prolonged immobilization.

17. IV nitroglycerin should be continued x 24-48 hours for large anterior MI, heart failure, hypertension, or recurrent ischemia.

18. Stress testing is performed in low- and intermediate-risk patients without rest pain or heart failure after a minimum of 12-24 hours and 2-3 days, respectively. If baseline ECG abnormality precludes assessment of ST-segment shifts (e.g., LBBB, LVH with repolarization changes), an exercise test with radionuclide imaging is recommended. Patients unable to exercise should undergo a pharmacological stress test.

19. High-risk findings include any of the following: 2nd troponin positive at 4-8 hours; repeat ECG shows ischemic ST-T changes; recurrent rest angina; recurrent exertional angina with heart failure or mitral regurgitation; LVEF < 0.40; hemodynamic instability; sustained ventricular tachycardia; prior PCI within 6 months; prior CABG; or high-risk noninvasive test result (> 3% annual mortality): rest or exercise LVEF < 0.35; treadmill score ≤ −11; single large stress-induced perfusion defect or multiple moderate perfusion defects; large fixed perfusion defect or moderate stress-induced perfusion defect with LV dilatation or thallium uptake in lung; echo wall motion abnormality > 2 segments with low-dose dobutamine (< 10 mcg/kg/min) or at a low heart rate (< 120 bpm); or extensive ischemia on stress echo.

20. Secondary prevention measures include aspirin, beta-blocker, ACE inhibitor, statin, exercise, smoking cessation, weight control, Mediterranean diet. Consider gemfibrozil for low HDL cholesterol and fish oil (omega-3) supplement. Control hypertension (blood pressure ≤ 130/85 mmHg), diabetes mellitus (HgbA1c < 7%), and dyslipidemia (LDL cholesterol ≤ 100 mg/dL; HDL-cholesterol > 40 mg/dL; triglyceride ≤ 150

mg/dL). Provide instructions to patient and family on the use of nitrates for recurrent pain, when to return to the emergency room, the purpose and dose of each discharge medication, and the importance of compliance.

Early Management of Non-ST-Elevation ACS Based on Risk Category (Figure 7.1, Table 7.1)

A. **High-Risk Patients.** These patients are best treated with early (< 12-48 hours) catheterization followed by PCI (in conjunction with a GP IIb/IIIa inhibitor and antithrombin therapy) or CABG based on anatomy. Clinical trials have shown benefit for abciximab,[136,137] eptifibatide,[138-140] and tirofiban.[141-143] In TARGET, the only head-to-head comparison of GP IIb/IIIa inhibitors to date, abciximab was superior to tirofiban at reducing the 30-day composite endpoint of death, MI, or urgent target vessel revascularization in ACS patients undergoing PCI (6.3% vs. 9.3%, p = 0.002).[144] GP IIb/IIIa inhibitors can be administered several hours prior to PCI, which may be of particular benefit when PCI will be delayed ≥ 12-24 hours (Table 8.2, p. 74), or at the start of the procedure. All high-risk patients without contraindications should also receive aspirin, clopidogrel, and a beta-blocker. Clopidogrel should be withheld 5-7 days prior to CABG. Since it is difficult to know if a patient will require CABG until angiography has been performed, and since many practices currently use early (< 24 hours) angiography in such patients, some advocate withholding clopidogrel until the coronary anatomy is defined.[85] (See pp. 77-78.)

B. **Intermediate-Risk Patients.** Patients with prior PCI or CABG should be treated the same as high-risk patients. Other intermediate-risk patients can be managed by the early invasive or early conservative approach to revascularization (Table 7.1). Early conservative management consists of a GP IIb/IIIa inhibitor (eptifibatide or tirofiban) plus antithrombin therapy (subcutaneous enoxaparin or IV unfractionated heparin), followed by late angiography and revascularization for any of the following: elevated cardiac markers or ischemic ECG changes on repeat testing; recurrent rest angina; exertional angina with heart failure or mitral regurgitation; LV dysfunction (EF < 0.40); high-risk noninvasive stress test result; hemodynamic instability; or sustained VT. High-risk (> 3% annual mortality) findings on noninvasive testing include rest or exercise LVEF < 0.35, treadmill score ≤ -11, single large or multiple moderate stress-induced perfusion defects,

Table 7.1.   Approach to Revascularization for Non-ST-Elevation ACS

Risk Category*	Approach**
High-risk	Early invasive approach
Intermediate-risk	
Prior PCI or CABG	Early invasive approach
All other	Early invasive or early conservative approach
Low-risk	Early conservative approach or manage as outpatient+

*   See Table 6.2, p. 62, for description of risk categories.

** Early invasive approach: early (within 12-24 hours) angiography and revascularization (PCI or CABG). Early conservative approach: angiography and revascularization for recurrent ischemia, LV dysfunction (EF < 0.40), or high-risk finding on stress test.

+   Low-risk patients with normal troponin levels on repeat testing, stable ECGs, no further ischemia, and a normal echocardiogram or stress test during observation in the emergency department may be considered for outpatient management similar to patients with chronic stable angina. Stress testing is recommended within 48-72 hours if not performed in the emergency department prior to discharge.

fixed perfusion defect with LV dilatation or thallium uptake in lung, and stress echo demonstrating extensive ischemia or echo wall motion abnormality in ≥ 2 myocardial segments with low-dose dobutamine (< 10 mcg/kg/min) or at low heart rate (< 120 bpm).[145] All intermediate-risk patients without contraindications should receive aspirin, clopidogrel, and a beta-blocker. Clopidogrel should be withheld for 5-7 days prior to CABG.

C. **Low-Risk Patients.** Patients with new-onset or progressive angina without prolonged (> 20 min) chest pain or other intermediate- or high-risk features should be triaged to PCI for the same indications as intermediate-risk patients (p. 67). For asymptomatic, low-risk patients without ST-T changes or elevated cardiac troponins, one approach is to follow these patients in the emergency department for 8-12 hours and consider discharge to home if repeat serum cardiac troponins are negative, serial ECGs remain stable, 2D echo (or possibly stress test) is normal, and there is no further evidence of ischemia. Discharged patients are managed on an outpatient basis similar to patients with chronic stable angina; a stress test is recommended within 72 hours if not performed during observation in the emergency department.

Hospital Management

Aspirin, clopidogrel, and beta-blockers are continued throughout hospitalization. For patients initially triaged to PCI, a GP IIb/IIIa inhibitor and heparin are given at the start of the case and continued for up to 24 hours after PCI (Table 9.3, p. 83). For patients triaged to early conservative management, eptifibatide or tirofiban is given for 48-96 hours, and UFH or enoxaparin is continued for 2-5 days. If PCI becomes necessary, eptifibatide or tirofiban should be continued for 18-24 hours post-intervention; it is not necessary to switch to abciximab for PCI. Patients scheduled for CABG are usually switched from enoxaparin to UFH prior to surgery, and clopidogrel is withheld 5-7 days prior to surgery, if possible. All patients with acute MI should receive an oral ACE inhibitor after urgent PCI (if performed) and once blood pressure has stabilized, usually no sooner than 6 hours, starting at a low dose and titrated upward. Analgesics and anxiolytics are prescribed as needed, stool softeners are given to all patients, and IV nitroglycerin, prolonged heparin therapy, and calcium antagonists are considered for special patient populations (Table 3.4, p. 32). Vital signs should be assessed every 30 minutes until stable, then every 4 hours, and pulse oximetry is usually monitored for at least one day. Bed rest with bedside commode is recommended for 12 hours, followed by a progressive increase in activity, as tolerated. Patients should be kept NPO until pain free, then advanced to clear liquids, and then to a low saturated fat diet. Frequent assessment for mechanical, ischemic, and electrical complications (e.g., heart failure, acute mitral regurgitation, VSD, reinfarction, arrhythmias, heart block) is mandatory. Stress testing and echocardiography (or radionuclide ventriculography) are recommended to identify residual ischemia and assess LV function, respectively, but are not routinely performed after successful PCI. Electrophysiology testing is recommended for VF or sustained VT $\geq$ 2 days post-MI and for nonsustained VT $\geq$ 4 days post-MI in patients with LV dysfunction (EF < 0.40).

Post-Discharge Measures

Therapeutic lifestyle changes and other secondary prevention measures are the same as for ST-elevation MI (p. 30).

Chapter 8

Interventional Management of
Non-ST-Elevation ACS

Early Invasive vs. Early Conservative
Approach to Revascularization

Four randomized trials of non-ST-elevation ACS have compared early invasive management (routine angiography and revascularization) to early conservative management (angiography and revascularization for recurrent ischemia) (Table 8.1).

A. **Early Trials (TIMI-3B,[146] VANQWISH [147]).** These trials showed no difference (TIMI-3B) or increased risk (VANQWISH) of death or MI with early routine revascularization. However, in TIMI-3B, PTCA resulted in earlier discharge, fewer readmissions, and less need for antianginal medication. Furthermore, 40% of the "conservatively treated" patients required revascularization.[146] In VANQWISH, the higher rate of in-hospital death or MI was primarily due to the high (10.4%) surgical mortality rate in the invasive group.[147] There were also marked delays (8 days) prior to revascularization, low (21%) rates of PTCA or CABG in the invasive group, and patients at "very high risk" (i.e., those most likely to benefit the most from revascularization) were excluded from VANQWISH. Importantly, these trials were performed prior to the availability of stents and GP IIb/IIIa inhibitors, limiting their relevance to current practice.

B. **FRISC-2.** In this trial, 2457 patients < 75 years old with non-ST-elevation ACS and no prior CABG were randomized to an early invasive or early conservative strategy. If possible, patients were also treated with low-molecular-weight heparin (dalteparin) for 4-5 days prior to angiography. Stents were used in 61% of cases. At 1 and 2 years, patients randomized to the early invasive strategy had less death, less MI, and less need for revascularization procedures (Table 8.1).[148,148b]

Table 8.1.   Early Invasive vs. Early Conservative Approach to Non-ST-Elevation ACS*

Trial	N	Outcomes	Comments
		Invasive vs. Conservative	
RITA-3 (2002)[148a]	1810	Death, MI, or refractory angina at 4 months (9.6% vs. 14.5%, p = 0.001), mainly due to a halving of refractory angina. No difference in death or MI between groups	Angiography was performed within 48 hours. Enoxaparin was the antithrombin in both groups. Discretionary use of GP IIb/IIIa inhibitors. Invasive approach resulted in less angina and fewer antianginal meds at follow-up
FRISC II (2002)[148,148b]	2457	1-year death (2.2% vs. 3.9%, p = 0.016), MI (8.6% vs. 11.6%, p = 0.015), death or MI (10.4% vs. 14.1%, p = 0.005); 2-year death (3.7% vs. 5.4%, p = 0.038), MI (9.2% vs. 12.7%, p = 0.005), death or MI (12.1% vs. 16.3%, p = 0.003)	In ACS patients treated with dalteparin (avg. 6 days prior to angiography), the invasive approach demonstrated clear benefit at 6 months, 1 year, and 2 years. Most PCI patients underwent coronary stenting
TACTICS-TIMI 18[149] (2001)	2220	6-month death, MI, or readmission for ACS (15.9% vs. 19.4%, p = 0.025); 6-month death or MI (7.3% vs. 9.5%, p < 0.05). Similar benefit in men and women[149a]	In ACS patients treated with tirofiban (avg. 22 hours prior to angiography), the early invasive approach was superior to the early conservative approach. Most PCI patients underwent coronary stenting
VANQWISH[147] (1998)	920	Hospital death (4.5% vs. 1.3%, p = 0.007), death or MI (7.8% vs. 3.3%, p = 0.004); 1-year death (12.6% vs. 7.9%, p = 0.025), death or MI (24% vs. 18.6%, p = 0.05)	High mortality rate in the invasive group was due to unusually high (10.4%) 30-day mortality after CABG. Most PCI patients underwent PTCA

ACS = acute coronary syndrome, LOS = length of stay, MI = myocardial infarction, PCI = percutaneous coronary intervention, PTCA = percutaneous transluminal coronary (balloon) angioplasty, TVR = target vessel revascularization

*   Early invasive approach = routine angiography and revascularization as appropriate; early conservative approach = angiography and revascularization for recurrent ischemia or high-risk finding on stress test

Table 8.1.   Early Invasive vs. Early Conservative Approach to Non-ST-Elevation ACS* (cont'd)

Trial	N	Outcomes Invasive vs. Conservative	Comments
TIMI-3B[146] (1994)	1473	Hospital death (2.4% vs. 2.5%, p = NS), MI (5.1 vs. 5.7%, p = NS), LOS (10.2 days vs. 10.9 days, p = 0.01); 6-week death (2.5% vs. 2.4%, p = NS), MI (5.7% vs. 5.1%, p = NS)	At 6 weeks, the invasive approach resulted in less readmission (7.8% vs 14.1%, p = 0.001) and less need for > 2 antianginals (44% vs. 52%, p = 0.02). Invasive group also had a shorter LOS. Most PCI patients underwent PTCA

ACS = acute coronary syndrome, LOS = length of stay, MI = myocardial infarction, PCI = percutaneous coronary intervention, PTCA = percutaneous transluminal coronary (balloon) angioplasty, TVR = target vessel revascularization

*   Early invasive approach = routine angiography and revascularization as appropriate; early conservative approach = angiography and revascularization for recurrent ischemia or high-risk finding on stress test

C.   TACTICS-TIMI 18.[143]   Recently, 2220 patients with non-ST-elevation ACS treated with aspirin, heparin, beta-blockers, and tirofiban on admission to the hospital were randomized to an early invasive strategy (routine catheterization within 48 hours followed by revascularization as appropriate) or an early conservative strategy (catheterization for recurrent ischemia or abnormal stress test). Stents were used in > 80% of cases. The primary endpoint of death, MI, or rehospitalization for ACS at 6 months was reduced by 18% in the invasive group (15.9% vs 19.4%, p = 0.025), with greatest benefit among high- and intermediate-risk patients. For patients with elevated troponin levels, early invasive management resulted in a 10% absolute reduction and a 39% relative reduction in the primary endpoint at 6 months (p < 0.001). In contrast, there was no advantage to early PCI in low-risk patients with normal cardiac troponins. The 4.7% rate of death or nonfatal MI at 30 days in the early invasive group is the lowest event rate reported in any ACS trial. Preprocedural (upstream) use of tirofiban (average 22 hours before PCI) appeared to prevent the increased risk of acute MI observed prior to PCI in FRISC-2 and other trials.

Stents vs. PTCA

In more than 7000 patients with unstable angina treated with stents or PTCA, stents resulted in fewer in-hospital ischemic complications, including less death (1.5% vs. 2.6%, p = 0.003), recurrent angina (23.5% vs. 47.4%, p < 0.00001), Q-wave MI (0.4% vs. 1.9%, p < 0.00001), repeat PTCA (13.8% vs. 30.6%, p < 0.00001), and CABG (6.5% vs. 19.6%, p < 0.00001), but there was no difference in mortality at 1 year.[149] Further benefit on restenosis (but probably not death or MI) is likely to be achieved with drug-eluting stents which, in early trials, have led to 50-90% reductions in clinical and angiographic restenosis compared to standard stents (Table 4.3, p. 35).

GP IIb/IIIa Inhibitors and PCI

Data support the routine use of abciximab, eptifibatide, or tirofiban in patients with non-ST-elevation ACS being treated with PCI, particularly those with elevated cardiac troponin levels or dynamic ST-segment changes.[136-143] As adjuncts to aspirin, heparin, and beta-blockers, GP IIb/IIIa inhibitors reduce the risk of major adverse cardiac events after PCI by 30-40% (Table 9.2, p. 82). Only abciximab has shown long-term (> 1 year) mortality benefit in stent patients;[136-150] eptifibatide reduced the rate of death or MI at 1 year in ESPRIT, but mortality benefit did not reach statistical significance.[138] In TARGET, the only head-to-head comparison of GP IIb/IIIa inhibitors as adjuncts to PCI, abciximab reduced the risk of MI at 30 days (5.8% vs. 8.5%, p = 0.004) and 6 months (7.2% vs. 8.8%, p = 0.013) in ACS patients compared to tirofiban, but 6-month mortality rates were the same in both groups (1.39%).[144] Results from PURSUIT (eptifibatide),[140] PRISM-PLUS (tirofiban),[151] and CAPTURE (abciximab)[137] suggest that upstream (pre-interventional) administration of GP IIb/IIIa inhibitors can reduce the risk of acute MI prior to PCI by up to 70% (Table 8.2). The optimal timing of GP IIb/IIIa inhibitors in relation to PCI awaits determination.

**Table 8.2. GP IIb/IIIa Inhibitors and Acute MI in Patients Awaiting
PCI for Non-ST-Elevation ACS**

		Incidence of MI Prior to PCI (%)		
Trial	GP IIb/IIIa Inhibitor	GP IIb/IIIa Inhibitor	Control	p-Value
PURSUIT[140]	Eptifibatide	1.8	5.5	0.001
PRISM-PLUS[151]	Tirofiban	0.8	2.4	0.01
CAPTURE[137]	Abciximab	0.6	2.1	0.29

Coronary Artery Bypass Grafting (CABG)

CABG is the preferred method of revascularization for patients with ACS and
either significant left main obstruction or LV dysfunction (or possibly treated
diabetes) plus 3-vessel disease or 2-vessel disease with proximal LAD
involvement. Since the risks of perioperative death (4%) and acute MI (10%) are
high when CABG is performed on an urgent basis, efforts should be made to
stabilize patients pharmacologically and, if needed, with IABP counterpulsation
prior to surgical revascularization.

Recommendations

The current weight of evidence favors early (< 12-48 hours) coronary stenting
plus abciximab or eptifibatide for patients with non-ST-elevation ACS at high-
risk of thrombotic complications (e.g., elevated troponins, dynamic ST-segment
changes), in conjunction with aspirin, clopidogrel, heparin, and beta-blockers.
For anticipated delays in PCI > 24 hours, it is reasonable to begin eptifibatide,
but not abciximab, immediately on admission and to continue it for 18-24 hours
post-PCI. Technical considerations are similar to PCI for ST-elevation MI:
stenting is usually performed on the culprit vessel to achieve a residual stenosis
< 30% and TIMI-3 flow. Hospitalized patients at lower risk of thrombotic
complications can be managed medically with aspirin, clopidogrel, beta-
blockers, heparin, and eptifibatide or tirofiban and later triaged to
angiography/revascularization for failed medical therapy or high-risk results on
noninvasive testing.

Chapter 9

Antiplatelet and Antithrombin Therapy for Non-ST-Elevation ACS

Aspirin

A. **Overview.** Aspirin is a salicylic acid derivative that exerts its antiplatelet effects by blocking the formation of thromboxane A_2 through irreversible acetylation of platelet cyclooxygenase. This effect is transient in nucleated cells but is permanent for the 10-day lifespan of anucleate platelets. Aspirin reduces the risk of death, MI, or stroke by 29% at 1 month following acute MI and by 36% at 6 months following unstable angina.[152] Aspirin also reduces the risk of abrupt coronary occlusion after PCI by 50-75%[153,154] and helps maintain saphenous vein graft patency after CABG.[155] However, aspirin increases the risk of bleeding, has no impact on restenosis after PCI,[156] and does not prevent platelet adhesion or platelet aggregation in response to thrombin, catecholamines, ADP, serotonin, or shear-stress. Up to 10% of patients with coronary artery disease are aspirin-resistant.[157]

B. **Dose.** All patients should immediately receive 2-4 chewable nonenteric-coated baby aspirins (81 mg each), as buccal absorption of chewed aspirin is the fastest route for platelet inhibition. The initial dose should be followed by 75-325 mg of an enteric or nonenteric preparation (PO) q24h long term. Rectal suppositories (325 mg) can be used for patients unable to take oral medications. Enteric-coated preparations should be avoided acutely due to delays in GI absorption and antiplatelet effects.

Clopidogrel

A. **Overview.** Clopidogrel is an inhibitor of ADP-induced platelet aggregation acting by direct inhibition of ADP binding to its receptor and of the subsequent ADP-mediated activation of the platelet GP IIb/IIIa complex. This results in platelet inhibition to a broad range of platelet agonists. Clopidogrel irreversibly modifies the platelet ADP receptor, so that platelets exposed to clopidogrel are affected for the remainder of their lifespan. Compared to ticlopidine, another thienopyridine derivative, clopidogrel has a longer duration of action, faster onset of action, and is better tolerated with fewer adverse hematologic effects.[158-161]

B. **Use in Non-ST-Elevation ACS**
   1. **Primary Medical Therapy.** The role for dual antiplatelet therapy with aspirin and clopidogrel was recently evaluated in the CURE trial.[162] In this study, 12,562 patients with unstable angina or non-ST-elevation MI were treated with aspirin (75-325 mg PO q24h) and randomized to clopidogrel (300 mg loading dose followed by 75 mg/day) or placebo for 3-12 months (average 9 months). Patients treated with GP IIb/IIIa inhibitors within 3 days or revascularization within 3 months were excluded from this study as were patients scheduled for the aggressive interventional approach to ACS. As shown in Table 9.1, clopidogrel resulted in a highly significant 20% reduction in the primary composite endpoint of cardiovascular death, MI, or stroke (9.3% vs. 11.5%, p < 0.001). There was a 1% absolute increase in major bleeding complications with clopidogrel, but these cases were effectively managed by blood transfusions, and there was no increase in fatal bleeding. Major bleeding within 7 days after surgery was increased by 53% when clopidogrel was discontinued within 5 days of CABG surgery (9.6% vs. 6.3%), but there was no significant increase in bleeding when clopidogrel was stopped 5 days or more prior to surgery. Based on CURE, the ACC/AHA Guideline Update from March, 2002, recommends that clopidogrel should be added to aspirin as soon as possible on admission and continued for at least 1 month and possibly for 9 months for non-ST-elevation ACS patients in whom a non-interventional approach is planned.[128]

Table 9.1. Dual Antiplatelet Therapy for Non-ST-Elevation ACS: Results of the CURE Trial[162]

Endpoint (avg. 9 months)	Aspirin (n = 6303)	Aspirin + Clopidogrel (n = 6259)	Risk Ratio	p-Value
CV death, MI, or stroke (%)*	11.5	9.3	0.80	< 0.001
CV death, MI, stroke, or refractory ischemia (%)	19.0	16.7	0.88	0.0004
Major bleeding (%)	2.7	3.6	1.34	0.003
Minor bleeding (%)	8.6	15.3	1.78	< 0.001

ACS = acute coronary syndromes; CURE = Clopidogrel in Unstable angina to prevent Recurrent Events; CV = cardiovascular; MI = myocardial infarction
* Primary endpoint

2. **Adjunct to PCI**. 2658 of 12,562 patients in CURE underwent PCI. Patients received study drug (clopidogrel or placebo) for a median of 10 days prior to PCI, then open-label clopidogrel for 2-4 weeks after PCI, then resumption of study drug for a mean of 8 months. Clopidogrel resulted in an overall (before and after PCI) reduction in cardiovascular death or MI by 31% (8.8% vs. 12.6%, p = 0.002).[163] Although not a prespecified endpoint, clopidogrel did not increase the risk of major or life-threatening bleeding in patients receiving GP IIb/IIIa inhibitors. Based on PCI-CURE, the ACC/AHA Guideline Update from March, 2002, recommends that clopidogrel should be added to aspirin for at least 1 month and possibly for 9 months in PCI patients not at high risk of bleeding.[128] Clopidogrel should be withheld 5-7 days prior to CABG.

3. **Unresolved Issues.** Additional studies are required to assess the safety and efficacy of triple antiplatelet therapy with aspirin, clopidogrel, and GP IIb/IIIa inhibitors for primary medical therapy of ACS. Because of this unresolved issue, one of three strategies is reasonable: (1) Initiate a GP IIb/IIIa inhibitor (small molecule eptifibatide or tirofiban) in high-risk patients and reserve clopidogrel until the coronary anatomy is visualized and a decision is made to proceed with PCI. Use immediate clopidogrel in low-risk patients not eligible for a GP IIb/IIIa inhibitor;

(2) Initiate both clopidogrel and a GP IIb/IIIa inhibitor in high-risk patients and clopidogrel alone in low-risk patients; (3) Initiate clopidogrel in all patients and withhold the GP IIb/IIIa inhibitor until the anatomy is visualized and a decision is made to proceed with PCI. Based on the preponderance of data, it is now our preference to initiate both clopidogrel and a GP IIb/IIIa inhibitor in high-risk patients as soon as possible.

C. **Other Uses for Clopidogrel**
   1. **Coronary stenting.** Numerous randomized trials have confirmed the superiority of dual antiplatelet therapy compared with aspirin alone or aspirin plus warfarin at reducing ischemic events after coronary stenting. In the randomized CLASSICS trial of 1020 patients undergoing elective stenting,[164] clopidogrel was better tolerated than ticlopidine, and in an analysis of 8 randomized trials or registries, clopidogrel resulted in fewer major adverse cardiac events than ticlopidine.[125]
   2. **Secondary prevention.** Clopidogrel proved somewhat more effective than aspirin for secondary prevention in CAPRIE, in which 19,185 patients with MI within 35 days, ischemic stroke within 6 months, or symptomatic peripheral arterial disease were randomized to clopidogrel (75 mg/d) or aspirin (325 mg/d) for 1-3 years.[166] At 1.6 years, clopidogrel reduced the composite endpoint of new ischemic stroke, new MI, or other vascular death by 8.7% relative to aspirin (5.32% vs. 5.83%, p = 0.043). Benefit was greatest in patients with peripheral arterial disease. Aspirin resulted in slightly more gastrointestinal bleeding compared with clopidogrel, and there was no difference in the incidence of severe neutropenia (0.1%).

D. **Safety Profile.** The safety profile of clopidogrel is similar to that of low-dose aspirin, with a rare incidence of thrombotic thrombocytopenic purpura (TTP). The most frequent side effects include diarrhea, rash, and pruritus.[161] Clopidogrel is not associated with an increased risk of neutropenia, so routine hematologic monitoring is not necessary for patients on chronic therapy. One report documented 11 cases of TTP among 3 million patients exposed to clopidogrel,[167] although the incidence of TTP is substantially lower than that associated with ticlopidine.[168] Due to an increased risk of perioperative bleeding, clopidogrel should be discontinued for 5-7 days prior to CABG. Clopidogrel is metabolized in the liver but has little impact on hepatic enzyme induction or drug metabolism

Platelet Glycoprotein (GP) IIb/IIIa Receptor Antagonists

A. **Overview.** Activation of the platelet GP IIb/IIIa receptor complex is a critical event in the pathogenesis of arterial thrombosis and ACS. GP IIb/IIIa receptor antagonists represent a major breakthrough as adjuncts to PCI and in the medical management of high-risk patients.

B. **Mechanism of Action.** GP IIb/IIIa inhibitors prevent platelets from binding to fibrinogen via the GP IIb/IIIa receptor, the final obligatory pathway for platelet aggregation (Figure 9.1).[169,170] GP IIb/IIIa inhibitors are the most potent antiplatelet agents available, blocking platelet aggregation in response to all platelet agonists (e.g., collagen, thrombin, ADP, epinephrine, thromboxane A_2). They do not, however, prevent platelet adhesion or the formation of thrombin, fibrin, or coagulation factors.

C. **Impact on Prognosis**. In more than 48,000 patients enrolled in 14 large-scale, randomized, placebo-controlled trials, GP IIb/IIIa inhibitors resulted in significant reductions in the relative risk of death or MI at 30 days when used as an adjunct to PCI (36% reduction) or as primary medical therapy for ACS (9% reduction) (Table 9.2). Higher-risk patients derived the most benefit, especially those with elevated cardiac troponin levels.[15,170a]

D. **Types of Inhibitors (Table 9.3).** Two intravenous GP IIb/IIIa inhibitors (eptifibatide, tirofiban) have been approved for use in ACS; abciximab may be used in ACS only when PCI is employed. Compared with competitive inhibitors (eptifibatide, tirofiban), noncompetitive inhibitors (abciximab) have longer biological half-lives, higher dissociation constants (resulting in more permanent binding), and more cross-reactivity with other cell-surface receptors.[171] Adjunctive antiplatelet and antithrombin therapy is described in Table 9.4.

   1. **Abciximab (ReoPro)**. Abciximab is the Fab fragment of the chimeric monoclonal antibody 7E3. In addition to GP IIb/IIIa inhibition, abciximab blocks the vitronectin receptor ($\alpha_v\beta_3$) on smooth muscle and endothelial cells and the MAC-1 receptor on leukocytes.[172,173] Abciximab also inhibits clot retraction, factor XIII, and PAI-I, displaces

fibrinogen, and prolongs the ACT, which may result in antiproliferative, anti-inflammatory, anticoagulant, and thrombolytic effects.

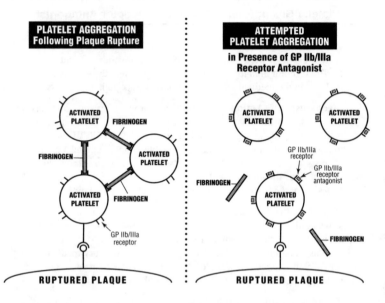

Figure 9.1. GP IIb/IIIa Receptor Antagonists and ACS

GP IIb/IIIa receptor antagonists are the most potent platelet inhibitors available. They exert their antiplatelet effects by blocking the binding of fibrinogen to the GP IIb/IIIa receptor on the platelet surface, the final common pathway of platelet aggregation. Abciximab is a monoclonal antibody and noncompetitive inhibitor that binds 1:1 to the GP IIb/IIIa receptor molecule to induce a conformational change that renders the fibrinogen-binding site of the receptor inactive. Eptifibatide and tirofiban are small-molecule competitive inhibitors of the RGD tripeptide-binding domain of the GP IIb/IIIa receptor.

2. **Eptifibatide (Integrilin).** Eptifibatide is a synthetic cyclic K-G-D (lysine-glycine-aspartic acid) heptapeptide.[174] In contrast to abciximab, eptifibatide is a competitive antagonist of the GP IIb/IIIa receptor, has a short half-life (2.5 hours),[175] and does not cross-react with the vitronectin receptor. Platelet function returns to baseline within 4-8 hours after drug discontinuation.[176]

3. **Tirofiban (Aggrastat).** Tirofiban is a synthetic small-molecule nonpeptide mimetic of the R-G-D (Arg-Gly-Asp) sequence of fibrinogen. Like eptifibatide, tirofiban is a competitive antagonist of the GP IIb/IIIa receptor, is rapidly reversible and highly selective, and does not cross-react with the vitronectin receptor.

E. **Indications in Non-ST-Elevation ACS.** GP IIb/IIIa inhibitors are indicated as adjuncts to PCI and as primary medical therapy for high-risk patients (e.g., elevated troponin or CK-MB levels, ST-segment depression or dynamic ST-segment shifts, prolonged refractory chest pain, hemodynamic instability).

F. **Safety Concerns.** A number of safety concerns have been raised about the use of GP IIb/IIIa inhibitors in general and about abciximab in particular, including bleeding complications, the potential requirement for emergency CABG, severe thrombocytopenia, and potential drug interactions. Virtually all of these considerations are readily prevented or treated and do not preclude the use of these agents.

1. **Bleeding.** In contrast to earlier abciximab trials using standard-dose heparin to maintain high ACT levels,[177] trials using low-dose heparin, early sheath removal, and target ACT levels of 200-250 seconds (EPILOG,[178] CAPTURE,[137] EPISTENT[136]) reported no difference in major or minor bleeding for patients treated with abciximab vs. placebo. These studies indicate that the risk of bleeding associated with abciximab can be minimized by low-dose heparin, early sheath removal, avoidance of venous sheaths, and fastidious post-procedure groin care. No GP IIb/IIIa inhibitor has been associated with an increased risk of intracranial hemorrhage.

Table 9.2 Meta-analysis of GP IIb/IIIa Inhibitor Trials

Study	IIb/IIIa Inhibitor	N	Death or MI at 30 Days (%) Placebo	Death or MI at 30 Days (%) GP IIb/IIIa
Percutaneous Coronary Intervention (ACS or Elective Indication)				
EPIC	Abciximab	2099	9.6	6.6
EPILOG	Abciximab	2792	9.1	4.0
EPISTENT	Abciximab	2399	10.2	5.2
RAPPORT	Abciximab	483	5.8	4.6
CAPTURE	Abciximab	1265	9.0	4.8
IMPACT II	Eptifibatide	4010	8.4	7.1
ESPRIT	Eptifibatide	2064	10.2	6.4
RESTORE	Tirofiban	2141	6.3	5.1
Total		**17,253**	**8.9**	**5.7**
Medical Therapy for Non-ST-Elevation ACS (Patients Not Scheduled for PCI)				
PARAGON A	Lamifiban	2282	11.7	11.3
PARAGON B	Lamifiban	5225	11.4	10.6
PRISM	Tirofiban	3231	7.1	5.8
PRISM-PLUS	Tirofiban	1570	12.0	8.7*
PURSUIT	Eptifibatide	10,948	15.7	13.4*
GUSTO-IV ACS	Abciximab	7800	8.0	8.2*
Total		**31,402**	**11.8**	**10.8**
All Studies		**48,655**	**10.8**	**9.0**

Fourteen large-scale, randomized, placebo-controlled trials of GP IIb/IIIa inhibitors. At 30 days, GP IIb/IIIa inhibitors reduced the composite endpoint of death or MI by 36% in PCI trials (p < 0.001), by 9% in trials of medical therapy for non-ST-elevation ACS (p = 0.015), and by 17% for all trials. Risk reduction was greatest for troponin-positive patients.
* Best dosage regimen selected for analysis.
Adapted from: Lancet 2002;359:189-98; Clev Clinic J Med 2000;67:131.

Table 9.3. GP IIb/IIIa Inhibitors for Non-ST-Elevation ACS

	Abciximab (ReoPro)	Eptifibatide (Integrilin)	Tirofiban (Aggrastat)
Description	Monoclonal antibody; noncompetitive inhibitor	Peptide; competitive inhibitor	Nonpeptide; competitive inhibitor
Duration of effect	24-48 hours after infusion	4-8 hours after infusion	4-8 hours after infusion
GP IIb/IIIa specificity	Cross-reacts with other receptors	Highly specific	Highly specific
GP IIb/IIIa binding	Permanent	Reversible	Reversible
Dose *Primary medical management (patients not scheduled for PCI)*	Not approved	**PURSUIT dose:** 180 mcg/kg IV bolus plus 2 mcg/kg/min IV infusion for up to 72-96 hours.* For arrival to the cath lab > 2 hours after initiating therapy, no additional bolus is required; otherwise, a second bolus of 180 mcg/kg is given	**PRISM-PLUS dose:** 0.4 mcg/kg/min IV loading infusion x 30 minutes plus 0.1 mcg/kg/min IV maintenance infusion for up to 48-96 hours. For CrCl < 30 cc/min, the infusion rate is reduced by 50%
Adjunct to PCI	0.25 mg/kg IV bolus at time of PCI plus 0.125 mcg/kg/min (max. 10 mcg/min) IV infusion x 12 hours. For patients with unstable angina scheduled for PCI within 24 hours, bolus plus infusion abciximab (PCI dose) can be started up to 24 hours prior to PCI and continued until 1 hour after the procedure	**ESPRIT dose:** 2 x 180 mcg/kg IV boluses, 10 minutes apart, at time of PCI plus 2 mcg/kg/min IV infusion x 18-24 hours*	**RESTORE/ TACTICS dose:** 10 mcg/kg IV bolus over 3 minutes immediately prior to PCI plus 0.15 mcg/kg/min IV infusion x 18-24 hours. For CrCl < 30 cc/min, the infusion rate is reduced by 50%

CrCl = creatinine clearance, PCI = percutaneous coronary intervention, UFH = unfractionated heparin. * For serum creatinine 2-4 mg/dL, reduce eptifibatide infusion to 1 mcg/kg/min.

Table. 9.4. Adjunctive Antithrombin and Antiplatelet Therapy for GP IIb/IIIa Inhibitors for Non-ST-Elevation ACS

Therapy	Dose
Heparin (unfractionated)	• As medical therapy in conjunction with a GP IIb/IIIa inhibitor: 60-70 U/kg IV bolus (max. 5000 U) plus 12-15 U/kg/min IV infusion (max. 1000 U/hr), adjusted to maintain aPTT at 1.5-2.5 times control (50-75 seconds) • As adjunct to PCI in conjunction with a GP IIb/IIIa inhibitor: 60 U/kg IV bolus to achieve intraprocedural ACT of 200-250 seconds. Higher heparin doses and target ACTs have been used with eptifibatide and tirofiban. No additional heparin is given after PCI
Enoxaparin (as alternative to UFH)*	• As primary medical therapy in conjunction with a GP IIb/IIIa inhibitor: 1 mg/kg SQ q12h x 2-8 days • As an adjunct to PCI in conjunction with a GP IIb/IIIa inhibitor: 0.75 mg/kg IV bolus. If patient has been treated with SQ enoxaparin and the last SQ dose < 8 hours, no additional enoxaparin is required; if last SQ dose > 8 hours, an additional 0.3 mg/kg IV should be given just before PCI
Aspirin/ clopidogrel	325 mg started at least 1 day prior to PCI followed by 75-325 mg PO q24h long term; for urgent PCI, give 4 chewable nonenteric-coated baby aspirins (325 mg total). For stent procedures, add clopidogrel 300 mg PO load followed by 75 mg PO q24h for at least 1 month and possibly for up to 9 months. (See pp. 76-78 for discussion on clopidogrel)

ACT = activated clotting time, ACS = acute coronary syndromes, PCI = percutaneous coronary intervention, UFH = unfractionated heparin
*   As an alternative to UFH, enoxaparin may be easier to administer and associated with better clinical outcomes (ASSENT-3, p. 55), but further testing will be needed before it is adopted widely.

2. **Thrombocytopenia.** The incidence of thrombocytopenia appears to be higher with abciximab than with eptifibatide or tirofiban. In abciximab trials, the incidence of mild thrombocytopenia (< 100,000/mm^3) was 2.6-5.6% and severe thrombocytopenia (< 50,000/mm^3) was 0.9-1.6%; platelet transfusions were needed in 1.6-5.5%. Unlike heparin-induced thrombocytopenia, abciximab-associated thrombocytopenia responds promptly to platelet transfusions (although severe thrombocytopenia

after abciximab retreatment may not respond as effectively).

3. **Emergency CABG**. The risk of bleeding during emergency CABG is increased in patients receiving abciximab plus heparin.[179,180] The hemostatic defect caused by abciximab is largely reversible with platelet transfusions, but the benefit is not immediate or complete. Key factors in reducing the risk of bleeding during emergency CABG include careful titration of heparin dose and liberal use of platelet transfusions, especially after coming off cardiopulmonary bypass. In contrast to abciximab, antiplatelet effects with eptifibatide or tirofiban usually resolve in 4-8 hours and platelet transfusions are ineffective. GP IIb/IIIa inhibitors should be discontinued prior to emergency CABG.

G. **Unresolved Issues.** Ongoing or planned trials will help determine the optimal GP IIb/IIIa inhibitor for non-ST-elevation ACS, including dose, duration, timing, and adjunctive use of antithrombin therapy (unfractionated heparin, low-molecular-weight heparin, direct thrombin inhibitors) and other antiplatelet agents (aspirin, clopidogrel). Among 746 high-risk non-ST-elevation ACS patients treated with eptifibatide and randomized to enoxaparin or UFH in the INTERACT trial, enoxaparin resulted in fewer major bleeding episodes at 96 hours (1.8% vs. 4.6%, p = 0.03) and less death or MI at 30 days (5% vs. 9%, p = 0.031).[197] The SYNERGY trial is randomizing 8000 patients with unstable angina being managed invasively to enoxaparin or unfractionated heparin.

Low-Molecular-Weight Heparin (LMWH)[181]

A. **Overview.** LMWHs are homogeneous glycosaminoglycans with a mean molecular weight of 4000-6000 formed by controlled enzymatic or chemical depolymerization of unfractionated heparin (UFH).[182,183] Enoxaparin has shown benefit over UFH for non-ST-elevation ACS in two randomized trials.

B. **LMWH vs. Unfractionated Heparin (Table 9.5)**
1. **Mechanism of Action.** LMWH and UFH inhibit clotting factors IIa (thrombin activity) and Xa (thrombin generation). LMWHs have more anti-Xa activity and less anti-IIa activity than UFH, and their anticoagulant effect, which is mediated primarily by inhibition of

thrombin generation, is not fully reflected in the aPTT (Figure 9.2).

2. **Ease of Use, Reliability of Anticoagulation, and Risk of Thrombocytopenia.** LMWHs have several advantages over UFH, including better inhibition of thrombin generation (higher anti-Xa:anti-IIa ratio), lack of need to monitor aPTT (due to enhanced bioavailability and a more reliable anticoagulant effect), ease of administration (reliable anticoagulation via subcutaneous route), lack of inhibition by platelet factor IV, and a lower risk of heparin-induced thrombocytopenia.[184] In clinical trials, LMWHs were associated with more minor bleeding than UFH, but there was no increase in major bleeding complications. Protamine is less effective at reversing the anticoagulant effects of LMWHs than UFH.

3. **Clinical Trials of LMWH for Non-ST-Elevation ACS (Table 9.6)**

   a. **Primary medical therapy (patients not scheduled for PCI).** Four major randomized trials compared LMWH to UFH as primary medical therapy for non-ST-elevation ACS (Table 9.6). A meta-analysis of 2 enoxaparin trials (ESSENCE,[185] TIMI 11b[186]) included a total of 7081 patients and showed a significant 20% reduction in the composite endpoint of death or MI at 8 days (4.1% vs. 5.3%, p = 0.02) and at 6 weeks (7.1% vs. 8.6%, p = 0.02) in favor of enoxaparin, without an increase in major bleeding complications.[187] At 1 year, enoxaparin reduced the risk of death, MI, or urgent revascularization compared to UFH by 12% (23.3% vs. 25.8%, p = 0.008).[188] In contrast, dalteparin (FRIC[189]) and nadroparin (FRAXIS[190]) had no impact on clinical outcome, suggesting important differences between LMWHs.[191]

   b. **Adjunct to PCI.** Since ACT and aPTT levels do not accurately reflect the degree of anticoagulation with LMWHs, UFH is preferred by most interventional cardiologists during PCI. However, recent observational studies (NICE-1, NICE-3, NICE-4)[192-194] and randomized trials (ACUTE II, CRUISE)[195-196] indicate that enoxaparin is a safe and effective alternative to UFH for procedural anticoagulation (with or without GP IIb/IIIa inhibitors), with similar rates of ischemic events and major bleeding complications.

Table 9.5. Comparison of Low-Molecular-Weight Heparin (LMWH) to Unfractionated Heparin (UFH)

	UFH	LMWH
Composition	Heterogeneous mixture of polysaccharides; molecular weight 3000-30,000	Homogeneous glycosaminoglycans; molecular weight 4000-6000
Mechanism of anticoagulation	Activates antithrombin; equivalent activity against factor IIa (thrombin) and factor Xa	Less activation of antithrombin; greater activity against factor Xa than factor IIa (thrombin); releases TFPI from endothelium
Pharmacokinetics	Variable binding to plasma proteins, endothelial cells, and macrophages results in unpredictable anticoagulant effects and short half-life	Minimal binding to plasma proteins, endothelial cells, and macrophages results in predictable anticoagulation and longer half-life
Laboratory monitoring	Essential because of unpredictable anticoagulant effects; monitor aPTT or ACT	Unnecessary except in renal failure or body weight < 45 kg or > 80 kg; monitor anti-factor Xa levels
Clinical uses	ACS; venous thrombosis; ischemic stroke. Routinely used during PCI. Preferred over LMWH for anticoagulation during CABG	At least as effective as UFH for non-ST-elevation ACS (enoxaparin may be better than UFH); venous thrombosis; ischemic stroke. At least as safe and effective as UFH during PCI with or without GP IIb/IIIa inhibitors
Neutralization	Protamine neutralizes antithrombin activity	Protamine neutralizes antithrombin activity but only partially reverses anti-factor Xa activity
HIT-2	Should not be used in patients with a history of HIT-2	Should not be used in patients with a history of HIT-2
Cost	Inexpensive	More expensive than unfractionated heparin, but costs are offset by lack of need for monitoring and fewer adverse events (enoxaparin)

ACS = acute coronary syndrome, CABG = coronary artery bypass graft surgery, HIT-2 = heparin-induced thrombocytopenia, TFPI = tissue factor pathway inhibitor

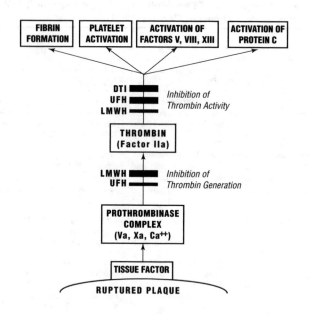

Figure 9.2. Antithrombin Therapy and ACS

Various antithrombins are used in clinical practice. Low-molecular-weight heparins (LMWH) and unfractionated heparin (UFH) bind factors Xa and IIa (thrombin) to reduce thrombin generation and thrombin activity, respectively. Direct thrombin inhibitors (DTI) (e.g., hirudin) reduce thrombin activity only. LMWHs have greater anti-Xa activity than UFH, resulting in greater inhibition of thrombin generation. Standard weight-adjusted dosing of LMWH produces a predictable level of anticoagulation, which is not fully reflected in the activated partial thromboplastin time (aPTT). Neither UFH nor LMWH bind clot-bound thrombin, in contrast to direct thrombin inhibitors. Since thrombin itself is a potent platelet activator, antithrombin agents also decrease platelet activation.

C. **Indications.** Enoxaparin is indicated as primary medical therapy for non-ST-elevation ACS to reduce the risk of death, MI, or target vessel revascularization. Contraindications include active major bleeding, thrombocytopenia with positive antiplatelet antibody tests, or hypersensitivity. Caution should be used in uncontrolled hypertension, diabetic retinopathy, serum creatinine < 30 cc/min, and in conditions associated with an increased risk of bleeding. UFH is preferred over LMWH in patients scheduled for CABG within 24 hours since the anticoagulant effects of UFH are more reliably reversed with protamine.

D. **Dose.** Enoxaparin 1 mg/kg SQ q12h x 2-8 days (median duration: ESSENCE trial 2.6 days;[185] TIMI 11b trial 4.6 days[186]). For PCI: 1 mg/kg IV if no GP IIb/IIIa inhibitor is used; 0.75 mg/kg IV if a GP IIb/IIIa inhibitor is used.

E. **Monitoring.** Platelet count (baseline, twice weekly), CBC, serum creatinine (baseline, change in renal function), and daily clinical evaluation for bleeding. The aPTT/ACT does not need to be monitored, as antithrombin activity is not fully reflected in these parameters.

F. **Complications**
    1. **Bleeding.** For significant bleeding warranting immediate reversal of anticoagulation, enoxaparin's anticoagulant effect can be partially reversed with protamine. Dosing is based on the time elapsed since the last enoxaparin dose:
        •   Last enoxaparin dose ≤ 8 hours: protamine 1 mg for each 1 mg of enoxaparin as a slow IV infusion. A second dose of 0.5 mg for each 1 mg of enoxaparin may be needed if the aPTT 2-4 hours after the first dose is prolonged.[198]
        •   Last enoxaparin dose > 8 hours but ≤ 12 hours: protamine 0.5 mg for each 1 mg of enoxaparin.
        •   Last enoxaparin dose > 12 hours: protamine may not be required.
    2. **Thrombocytopenia.** Enoxaparin should be discontinued if the platelet count drops below 100,000/mm³ or ≥ 50% from baseline.
    3. **Renal insufficiency.** Enoxaparin dose should be reduced by 25-50% in patients with significant renal impairment.

G. Recommendations and Unresolved Issues. Enoxaparin is recommended in conjunction with aspirin, clopidogrel, and GP IIb/IIIa inhibitors (in higher-risk patients) for primary medical management of non-ST-elevation ACS at a dose of 1 mg/kg SQ q12h x 2-8 days. UFH can also be used in this setting, but most data support the use of enoxaparin. Patients requiring PCI can be treated with enoxaparin or they can be switched to UFH to maintain an intraprocedural ACT of 300-350 seconds (or 200-250 seconds if a GP IIb/IIIa inhibitor is used). The ongoing SYNERGY trial is directly comparing enoxaparin and UFH in this setting. LMWH should be switched to UFH for anticoagulation during CABG.

Table 9.6. Clinical Trials of Low-Molecular-Weight Heparin vs. Unfractionated Heparin for Non-ST-Elevation ACS

Trial	LMWH	Design	Results (LMWH vs. UFH)
TIMI 11b[186] (1999)	Enoxaparin	3910 patients randomized to enoxaparin (30 mg IV bolus followed by 1 mg/kg SQ q12h) or UFH (70 U/kg IV bolus followed by 15 U/kg/hr IV infusion to maintain aPTT 1.5-2.5 times control) x 3-5 days (median duration: enoxaparin 4.6 days; UFH 3 days). Outpatient phase with re-randomization of UFH patients to enoxaparin or placebo x 6 weeks	Enoxaparin was superior to UFH at reducing death, MI, or urgent revascularization at 8 days (12.4% vs. 14.5%, p = 0.048) and at 43 days (17.3% vs. 19.6%, p = 0.048). No incremental benefit for outpatient enoxaparin. Minor bleeding was increased with enoxaparin, but not major bleeding
ESSENCE[18] (1997)	Enoxaparin	3171 patients randomized to enoxaparin (1 mg/kg SQ q12h) or UFH (5000 U IV bolus followed by an IV infusion to maintain aPTT at 55-86 sec.) x 2-8 days (median treatment 2.6 days)	Enoxaparin was superior to UFH at reducing death, MI, or recurrent angina at 14 days (19.8% vs. 23.3%, p = 0.019) and at 30 days (19.8% vs. 23.3%, p = 0.017)

Table 9.6. Clinical Trials of Low-Molecular-Weight Heparin vs. Unfractionated Heparin for Non-ST-Elevation ACS (cont'd)

Trial	LMWH	Design	Results (LMWH vs. UFH)
FRAXIS[190] (1999)	Nadroparin	3468 patients randomized to nadroparin (6 or 14 days) vs. UFH	No difference in death, MI, or refractory angina at 14 days (6-day nadroparin 17.8% vs. 14-day nadroparin 20.0% vs. UFH 18.1%) or at 3 months (22.3% vs. 22.3% vs. 26.2%). Trend toward increased death or MI in nadroparin group at all time points
FRIC[189] (1997)	Dalteparin	1482 patients randomized to dalteparin (120 IU/kg SQ q12h) or UFH x 6 days. At day 6 until day 45, second randomization to dalteparin (120 IU/kg SQ q24h) or placebo	No difference in death, MI, or recurrent angina (14% vs. 12.9%) or in bleeding (1.1% vs. 1%) at 45 days. Trend toward increased early risk of death, MI, or recurrent angina in dalteparin group (9.3% vs. 7.7% at 6 days, p = 0.33)

aPTT = activated partial thromboplastin time, IV = intravenous, MI = myocardial infarction, SQ = subcutaneous, UFH = unfractionated heparin

Direct Thrombin Inhibitors

Direct thrombin inhibitors are classified as polypeptide inhibitors (hirudin, bivalirudin) or low-molecular-weight inhibitors (argatroban).[199] In contrast to unfractionated heparin (UFH), hirudin and bivalirudin do not require antithrombin III for anticoagulant effect, form highly stable noncovalent complexes with circulating and clot-bound thrombin, and are not inhibited by platelet factor IV.[182] In a recent meta-analysis of 11 randomized trials comparing direct thrombin inhibitors with UFH for primary medical therapy of ACS or as adjuncts to PCI, direct thrombin inhibitors were associated with less death or MI at 1 week (4.3% vs. 5.1%, p = 0.001) and at 30 days (7.4% vs. 8.2%, p = 0.02).[200] Clinical benefit was observed for bivalent inhibitors (hirudin, bivalirudin) but not univalent inhibitors. The risk of major bleeding was increased with hirudin and decreased with bivalirudin. Bivalirudin is approved for procedural anticoagulation in unstable angina, and lepirudin (Refludan),[201] a recombinant hirudin, and argatroban (Acova) are approved for use in patients with heparin-induced thrombocytopenia who require IV anticoagulation. Lepirudin is administered as an initial bolus of 0.4 mg/kg (max. 44 mg) over 15-20 seconds followed by a continuous infusion of 0.15 mg/kg/hr (max. 16.5 mg/hr). The infusion rate should be reduced by 50%, 70%, and 85% for creatinine clearances of 45-60 mL/min, 30-44 mL/min, and 15-29 mL/min, respectively, and lepirudin should be avoided/discontinued if the creatinine clearance is < 15 mL/min. Argatroban is administered as a constant infusion of 2 mcg/kg/min (0.5 mcg/kg/min for patients with moderate hepatic impairment). Monitoring is accomplished using the same aPTT guidelines as for UFH. The role for direct thrombin inhibitors compared with LMWH or UFH awaits further definition.

HMG CoA-Reductase Inhibitors (Statins)[202]

Dyslipidemia is the most prevalent and important modifiable risk factor for atherosclerosis, affecting one in two U.S. adults. Proper treatment reduces the risk of acute MI and stroke by 25-80%, cardiovascular and all-cause mortality by 20-40%, and revascularization procedures by 22-30%. It has been estimated that for each 1% decrease in LDL cholesterol and each 1% increase in HDL cholesterol, the risk of cardiovascular events falls by 2% and 3%, respectively. Angiographic trials of statin therapy have consistently demonstrated increased regression of existing plaque and a reduction in the development of new atherosclerotic lesions. Despite marked benefits of lipid therapy, dyslipidemia is grossly undertreated: 80% of patients with coronary artery disease do not meet the LDL cholesterol targets established by the National Cholesterol Education Program Adult Treatment Panel III. Recent data suggest a role for in-hospital initiation of statins in ACS. In MIRACL, 3086 patients were randomized to atorvastatin 80 mg or placebo 1-4 days after admission for ACS. At 16 weeks, atorvastatin reduced the risk of death, MI, resuscitated cardiac arrest, or unstable angina by 16% (14.8% vs. 17.4%, p = 0.048).[203] Although the benefit was primarily due to a reduction in hospitalization for recurrent ischemia (as opposed to "hard" endpoints like death or MI), there was no apparent major harm associated with use of atorvastatin. A recent substudy from PRISM found that statin use for ≥ 30 days prior to the onset of ACS was associated with a 51% reduction in death or MI at 30 days, and that stopping statins in these patients was associated with a 3-fold increased risk of death or MI.[204] Given these results it is reasonable to initiate statin therapy at the time of hospitalization for ACS. Benefits to this approach include a potential reduction in early clinical events, a proven reduction in late clinical events, confirmed initiation of statin therapy, and improved patient compliance by linking statin therapy to the acute cardiac event. In CHAMP, in-hospital initiation of statins was associated with greater statin use at 1 year (91% vs. 10%) and a greater likelihood of having an LDL cholesterol level < 100 mg/dL (58% vs. 6%).[205] Recommendations regarding the choice of statin await the results of ongoing trials (A to Z trial, PROVE-IT, PACT).

Chapter 10

Special Patient Populations
and Non-ST-Elevation ACS

The management of non-ST-elevation ACS in women, diabetics, and post-CABG patients is similar to that of other ACS patients.[128] Special considerations are required in the very elderly, and nitrates and calcium antagonists are particularly useful for ACS secondary to variant (Prinzmetal's) angina or cocaine use (Table 10.1).

Table 10.1. Treatment of ACS in Special Patient Populations

Group	Treatment	Comments
Women	Treated similar to men	Women are older at presentation, have greater comorbidity, are more likely to present with atypical symptoms, and derive less benefit from GP IIb/IIIa inhibitors as primary medical therapy.[206] (Troponin-positive women given GP IIb/IIIa inhibitors derive benefit similar to troponin-positive men, but men are twice as likely to be troponin-positive than are women.) Hormone replacement therapy is not recommended for secondary prevention of cardiovascular events.[208] Cardiovascular disease causes more than twice the number of deaths as cancer, but < 10% of women perceive heart disease as their greatest threat.[207]
Age > 75 years	Intensity of management depends on overall general health. Enoxaparin and GP IIb/IIIa inhibitors improve outcomes	Elderly patients have greater comorbidity, more LV dysfunction, worse prognosis, and are more likely to manifest atypical symptoms. Baroreceptor sensitivity and cerebral autoregulation are often impaired, resulting in exaggerated hypotensive responses to nitrates and other vasodilators.

Table 10.1. Treatment of ACS in Special Patient Populations

Group	Treatment	Comments
Diabetics	Treated similar to non-diabetics. Tight glucose control is recommended	Diabetics have greater comorbidity, more extensive coronary disease, worse LV function, more silent ischemia, and worse prognosis after revascularization.[209,210] The risk of death in the first year after MI is 50%, half of which occurs before reaching the hospital. In BARI, diabetics with multivessel disease had better long-term outcomes after CABG vs. PTCA, but stents were not used in this study.[211]
Prior CABG	Treated similar to patients without CABG. Low threshold for angiography	CABG patients have more extensive coronary disease, worse LV function, more prior MI, and worse prognosis after ACS. Saphenous vein graft (SVG) plaques are often highly friable, ulcerated, and thrombotic.[212,213] PCI of acute SVG occlusions is associated with lower procedural success and higher early and late mortality compared to PCI of native vessel occlusions.[214,215]
Chest pain after cocaine use	Nitrates and calcium antagonists for ST-elevation or depression with ischemic chest pain.[216] Angiography for persistent ST-segment changes, and fibrinolytics (± PCI) for intracoronary thrombus[217,218]	Cocaine use increases the risk for coronary spasm and intravascular thrombosis.[219,220]
Variant (Prinzmetal's) angina	Nitrates, calcium antagonists, smoking cessation, PCI for obstructive CHD[221,222]	Provocative testing (e.g., ergonovine) should be considered in patients with non-obstructive coronary disease and transient ST-elevation during chest pain.

CABG = coronary artery bypass grafting, CHD = coronary heart disease, LV = left ventricular, MI = myocardial infarction, PCI = percutaneous coronary intervention,

Section 4

NON-MEDICAL THERAPY, MONITORING, RISK STRATIFICATION

Chapter 11. Non-Medical Therapy and Monitoring 97
Chapter 12. Risk Stratification 103

Chapter 11

Non-Medical Therapy and Monitoring Techniques

This section describes non-medical therapies and monitoring techniques used for the management of ACS. When used in conjunction with medical therapy, proper application of these modalities can reduce infarct size, preserve LV function, minimize ischemic, mechanical, and electrical complications, and improve survival.

Non-Medical Therapy and Monitoring Techniques for ACS

A. Transfer to Facility Equipped for PCI and CABG
   1. **Indications.** Lytic-ineligible patients with ST-elevation MI; persistent ischemia after fibrinolytic therapy; recurrent chest pain; hemodynamic instability (heart failure, hypotension, shock); suspected mechanical defect (VSD, acute MR); recurrent VT or VF that is difficult to control; possibly for lytic-eligible patients with ST-elevation MI (p. 41).
   2. **Comments.** The decision to transfer by ambulance or helicopter depends upon distance and driving time; for driving times > 120 minutes, helicopter transfer is recommended. During transfer, a paramedic or intensive care nurse should accompany the patient, and the ability to communicate by radio or phone with a physician is recommended. Arrhythmias, hypotension, and bleeding complications that develop during transfer can be treated effectively and are associated with low mortality rates.[47,49] Patients with non-ST-elevation MI may benefit from GP IIb/IIIa inhibitors prior to transfer.[222a]

B. Primary PCI
   1. **Indications.** ST-elevation MI; high-risk non-ST-elevation ACS; cardiogenic shock.
   2. **Comments.** Compared to fibrinolytic therapy for ST-elevation MI, primary PCI is associated with less reinfarction and recurrent ischemia, fewer strokes in high-risk patients, shorter hospital stay, and improved survival (Chapter 3). Stents are superior to PTCA, and routine use of

GP IIb/IIIa inhibitors is reasonable. For high-risk patients with non-ST-elevation ACS (e.g., elevated cardiac troponins, dynamic ST-segment changes, ongoing ischemia), an early invasive strategy plus a GP IIb/IIIa inhibitor is superior to an early conservative strategy of PCI for recurrent ischemia only (Chapter 8). Early revascularization (PCI or CABG) improves survival in cardiogenic shock (p. 135).

C. Immediate PCI After Successful Fibrinolysis (Patent Vessel)
  1. **Indications.** Continued or recurrent ischemia; hemodynamic instability or shock.
  2. **Comments.** Routine immediate PCI should not be performed on asymptomatic patients after successful fibrinolytic therapy. Compared to a conservative strategy, routine PTCA resulted in higher rates of emergency CABG and blood transfusions, similar reocclusion rates, no improvement in LV function, and a trend toward increased mortality.

D. Rescue PCI For Failed Fibrinolysis (Occluded Vessel)
  1. **Indications.** Ongoing chest pain; hemodynamic instability; persistent ST-elevation 60-120 minutes after starting fibrinolytic therapy, especially for large anterior MI; prior MI or impaired ventricular function in non-infarct zone.
  2. **Comments.** Rescue PTCA may improve clinical outcome and regional function of the infarct zone in high-risk patients with anterior MI.[223] Reocclusion rates are higher after rescue PTCA than after primary PTCA; therefore, stenting plus a GP IIb/III inhibitor is recommended to reduce the risk of reocclusion. When assessing the response to fibrinolytic therapy, the ECG lead with maximal ST-elevation at baseline should be evaluated for > 50% resolution (much more accurate and useful marker of persistent occlusion than persistent chest pain).

E. Delayed PCI (2-7 Days After Fibrinolysis)
  1. **Indications.** Spontaneous or inducible ischemia.
  2. **Comments.** Routine delayed PTCA should not be performed on asymptomatic patients with patent vessels. Compared to a conservative strategy of PTCA for recurrent ischemia, routine PTCA resulted in higher rates of abrupt closure, reinfarction, and urgent CABG, no improvement in LV function, and a trend toward increased mortality (Chapter 5). Late revascularization is recommended for recurrent ischemia and should be considered for high-risk patients with prior MI,

LV dysfunction, multivessel disease, or stenosis > 90% supplying a moderate or large area of myocardium. Patients with persistently occluded vessels that supply large myocardial territories should also be considered for delayed PCI since late patency may be important for infarct healing and the prevention of aneurysms and arrhythmias. This strategy is being tested in the NIH-sponsored OAT trial.

F. Coronary Artery Bypass Graft (CABG) Surgery

1. **Indications.** Failed PCI with ongoing ischemia or hemodynamic instability; left main disease; 3-vessel disease or 2-vessel disease with proximal LAD obstruction in the setting of LV dysfunction or treated diabetes; proximal 3-vessel disease with a patent infarct vessel, especially if unsuitable for PCI. Additional surgical procedures are required for ruptured papillary muscle, VSD, LV pseudoaneurysm, and free-wall rupture.

2. **Comments.** Perioperative mortality rates for elective CABG 3-7 days after acute MI are similar to other elective indications. Mortality rates are high for acute MI complicated by failed fibrinolytic therapy (13-17%), acute mitral regurgitation (27%-55%), or VSD (anterior MI 20%; posterior MI 70%). After fibrinolytic therapy, there is a 4% risk of reoperation for bleeding. BARI reported better outcomes with CABG vs. PTCA for patients with multivessel disease and treated diabetes,[211] but coronary stents and GP IIb/IIIa inhibitors were not tested in this trial. Compared to diabetics with prior PTCA, diabetics with prior CABG were more likely to survive spontaneous Q-wave MI.[224]

G. Intra-Aortic Balloon Pump (IABP) Counterpulsation

1. **Indications.** Cardiogenic shock not responding promptly to therapy; as a stabilizing bridge to surgical repair of ruptured chordae/papillary muscle or VSD; as a stabilizing bridge to revascularization for refractory post-infarct angina, significant left main disease, or critical 3-vessel disease with LV dysfunction, persistent ischemia, or hypotension.

2. **Comments.** IABP improves coronary perfusion via augmentation of diastolic blood pressure and improves cardiac output and lowers filling pressures via afterload reduction of the left ventricle. Routine use of IABP after successful primary PTCA has not been shown to improve outcome in high-risk or hemodynamically-stable patients.[225,226]

H. Temporary Pacemaker, *Prophylactic*

    1. Indications. Mobitz II 2° AV block; new LBBB; RBBB with left anterior or left posterior fascicular block (LAFB/LPFB); 1° AV block with RBBB or LBBB; alternating LBBB and RBBB; RBBB with alternating LAFB and LPFB.

    2. Comments. Prophylactic pacing (usually for 48-72 hours) is recommended to prevent hemodynamic collapse in the event that conduction delay progresses to complete heart block. Transcutaneous leads are preferred over transvenous leads because they can be applied quickly and used in standby mode for potentially unstable patients. Transcutaneous systems also avoid the risk of pneumothorax, cardiac perforation, and bleeding complications if anticoagulants/fibrinolytics are used. Nevertheless, a transvenous lead should be placed in patients who require more than brief transcutaneous pacing; are at high risk of progression to complete heart block; or develop asystole, complete heart block, or bradycardia with hypotension or recurrent sinus pauses > 3 seconds unresponsive to atropine.

I. Temporary Pacemaker, *Therapeutic* (Transvenous Lead Required)

    1. Indications. Asystole; 3° AV block; bradycardia with hypotension not responding to atropine; recurrent sinus pauses > 3 seconds not responding to atropine.

    2. Comments. Patients with hemodynamic instability may require transcutaneous pacing until a transvenous lead can be placed. Temporary pacing may not be required for 3° AV block that occurs with inferior MI and resolves with atropine. AV sequential pacing may be preferred over ventricular pacing to optimize AV synchrony ("atrial kick") and cardiac output in patients with severe LV dysfunction, LVH, or RV infarction. Frequent testing of pacing threshold is recommended; pacing energy is usually set at least 3 times threshold.

J. Permanent Pacemaker[227]

    1. Indications. Persistent 2° AV block in the His-Purkinje system accompanied by complete heart block or bilateral bundle branch block at any time during MI; bundle branch block with even transient Type II 2° AV block or complete heart block.

    2. Comments. Temporary pacing after acute MI is not by itself an indication for permanent pacing. Most of the excess mortality associated with high-grade conduction disturbances is caused by heart failure and ventricular arrhythmias from extensive myocardial necrosis, not progressive heart block.

K. Implantable Cardioverter-Defibrillator (ICD)

1. **Indications.** Sustained VT or VF > 48 hours from MI; nonsustained VT in post-MI patients with LV dysfunction and inducible VT at EP study; possibly for all patients with prior MI and severe LV dysfunction (EF < 0.30) based on MADIT-2.[230]

2. **Comments.**   In MADIT, patients with prior MI, EF < 36%, nonsustained VT, and inducible VT were randomized to ICD or best conventional therapy. At 4 years, the risk of death was reduced by 71% with prophylactic ICD (14% vs. 49%).[228] In MUSTT, ICDs were better than EP-guided drug therapy at reducing arrhythmic death in patients with coronary artery disease, nonsustained VT, and inducible VT during EP testing.[229] Most recently, in MADIT-2, 1232 patients with prior MI and severe LV dysfunction (EF ≤ 0.30) were randomized without EP testing to ICD or medical therapy. At 20 months, the risk of death was reduced by 31% with prophylactic ICD (14.2% vs. 19.8%, p = 0.016).[230] These data indicate significant survival benefit for ICD prophylaxis in patients with prior MI and LV dysfunction. Based on MADIT-2, there are 3-4 million potential ICD candidates now and 400,000 new candidates each year. Until further data can refine the population in which the ICD is indicated, the MADIT-2 criteria make a reasonable standard for ICD implantation.

L. Pulmonary Artery (PA) Catheterization

1. **Indications.** To differentiate cardiogenic shock from hypovolemic shock after failure of initial therapy with volume expansion or inotropic drugs. To guide management of cardiogenic shock, progressive hypotension, mechanical complications (VSD, papillary muscle rupture, cardiac tamponade), RV infarction with persistent hypotension or low cardiac output not responding to volume expansion and inotropes, and acute pulmonary edema not responding to diuretics, nitroglycerin, and inotropes.

2. **Comments.** PA catheterization allows determination of pulmonary capillary wedge pressure, cardiac output, and systemic vascular resistance. This information can be used to identify the etiology of

hypotension (e.g., hypovolemia, RV infarction, low cardiac output, acute VSD) and guide therapy in a variety of settings. PaO_2 measurements in the superior vena cava, right atrium, right ventricle, and pulmonary artery can be used to diagnose VSD and assess the severity of left-to-right shunting. Information obtained from PA catheterization (Table 11.1) and echocardiography with Doppler should be integrated into the decision making process for critically ill patients.

M. Intra-Arterial Pressure Monitoring

1. **Indications.** Severe hypotension (systolic BP < 80 mmHg) or cardiogenic shock; use of IV vasopressors or vasodilators (e.g., dopamine, sodium nitroprusside).

2. **Comments.** Monitoring via the radial artery is preferred, but the brachial or femoral artery can be used if needed. The intra-arterial catheter may remain in place at a single site up to 4 days as long as there is no evidence of thrombosis or infection, although in certain patients with difficult access it may be reasonable to leave the catheter in place longer.

Table 11.1. Pulmonary Artery Catheterization in ACS[231]

Complication	Usual Hemodynamic Findings
RV infarction	↑ RAP; RAP/PCWP ratio > 0.8; ↓ CO
Cardiogenic shock	↓ BP; ↓ CO; ↑ PCWP; ↑ SVR
Acute MR	↑ PCWP (prominent V-wave may be seen); CO usually ↓
Acute VSD	≥ 8% oxygen step-up from RA to RV/PA. CO calculations are falsely elevated (reflecting left-to-right shunting with increased pulmonary blood flow)
Cardiac tamponade	↓ BP; paradoxical pulse; RAP ~ PCWP; ↓ CO; prominent X-descent may be seen on RA tracing. May need echo to distinguish from RV infarction
Massive pulmonary embolism	↓ BP; ↓ CO; ↑ PA pressure and PVR; normal PCWP

BP = blood pressure, CO = cardiac output, MR = mitral regurgitation, PA = pulmonary artery, PCWP = pulmonary capillary wedge pressure, PVR = pulmonary vascular resistance, RA = right atrium, RAP = right atrial pressure, RV = right ventricular, SVR = systemic vascular resistance, VSD = ventricular septal defect

Chapter 12

Risk Stratification Post-MI

Predischarge risk stratification is indicated for all patients with ACS. As shown in Figure 12.1, if not performed early, cardiac catheterization is indicated to define coronary anatomy and assess LV function in patients with prior MI or CABG, known LV dysfunction, or a hospital course complicated by heart failure, hypotension, recurrent ischemia, failed fibrinolysis, suspected mechanical defect, or ventricular tachycardia or fibrillation > 48 hours from MI. All other patients should undergo stress testing, followed by cardiac catheterization for inducible ischemia, especially at low workloads (< 5 METS), or for other high-risk results (e.g., fixed perfusion defect with LV dilation or increased lung uptake of thallium, exercise-induced LV dysfunction or drop in systolic blood pressure). Guidelines for screening and evaluation of arrhythmias post-MI are proposed in Figure 12.2, although no approach is universally accepted. This section describes modalities used for risk stratification following acute MI.

Risk Stratification Modalities

A. **Stress Test**
   1. **Indications.** All patients not submitted for coronary angiography; select patients to assess functional capacity and the effectiveness of antianginal therapy.
   2. **Comments.** No single approach to exercise testing is universally accepted. One approach is to perform a submaximal stress test (70% of predicted maximal heart rate or up to 120-130 bpm) prior to discharge followed by a symptom-limited (maximal) stress test at 4-6 weeks. Another approach is to perform a symptom-limited stress test prior to discharge, which will identify a higher percentage of patients with residual ischemia compared to a submaximal test (40% vs. 23%).[232] Patients with resting ECG changes that preclude assessment of ST-segment shifts (e.g., LBBB, LVH with repolarization abnormality, ST

elevation or depression at rest) should undergo stress testing with radionuclide imaging. Patients unable to exercise should undergo a pharmacological stress test. Predictors of future cardiac events in patients who have not undergone reperfusion therapy include the inability to exercise 6 minutes, chest pain, ST-depression, hypotensive response to exercise, reversible thallium defects, thallium uptake in lung, and ≥ 5% fall in exercise ejection fraction. Stress testing is not routinely recommended following successful PCI.

B. Echocardiogram
 1. **Indications.** Heart failure; anterior MI; pericarditis; new murmur; sustained hypotension.
 2. **Comments.** Echocardiography can be used to assess LV function, evaluate the etiology of hypotension, and identify structural abnormalities post-MI (e.g., LV thrombus, aneurysm, pseudoaneurysm, pericardial effusion, RV infarction, ruptured papillary muscle). In conjunction with Doppler imaging, echocardiography can be used to identify acute mitral regurgitation and VSD.

C. Ambulatory (Holter) ECG Monitor
 1. **Indications.** Not routinely indicated. Obtain if patient is not on a computer-monitored telemetry system.
 2. **Comments.** Frequent VPCs or VT > 48 hours from MI identifies patients at increased risk of death. Implantable cardioverter-defibrillators (ICD) are beneficial for patients with low ejection fractions and inducible VT.[229]

D. Signal-Averaged ECG
 1. **Indications.** No clear indication. Possible utility for nonsustained VT > 48 hours from MI in patients with LV dysfunction (EF < 0.40).
 2. **Comments.** Signal-averaged ECG detects "late potentials" (i.e., areas of slowly conducted and fragmented electrical activity), which increase the risk of reentrant arrhythmias such as VT. If negative, the probability of inducing sustained monomorphic VT during EP testing is low. If positive, an EP study can be considered. The role and timing of the signal-averaged ECG are controversial.

E. Electrophysiology (EP) Study
 1. **Indications.** Sustained monomorphic VT > 48 hours from MI.

2. **Comments.** The utility of programmed electrical stimulation in post-MI patients remains controversial, as poor specificity results in many false positive tests. In MUSTT, there was no difference in outcome for patients with coronary artery disease and inducible VT treated by EP-guided medical therapy or no therapy; survival was greatest with ICD implantation.[229]

F. Cardiac Catheterization Post-MI

1. **Indications.** Recurrent ischemia; heart failure or hemodynamic instability; LV dysfunction (EF ≤ 0.40); new murmur with suspected mechanical defect; prior MI or CABG; VT > 48 hours from MI; inability to exercise; ischemia, arrhythmia, or fall in blood pressure during exercise testing.

2. **Comments.** Some advocate routine cardiac cath to eliminate the need for multiple costly noninvasive tests that subsequently indicate the need for catheterization in > 60% of patients with acute MI. Patients undergoing routine coronary angiography and revascularization based on coronary anatomy have low mortality rates (1% per year) after hospital discharge. Poor prognostic factors on cardiac catheterization include occluded infarct vessel or suboptimal flow, multivessel or left main disease, LV dysfunction (EF < 0.40), hypokinesis of non-infarct zone, and mechanical defects (acute mitral regurgitation, VSD).

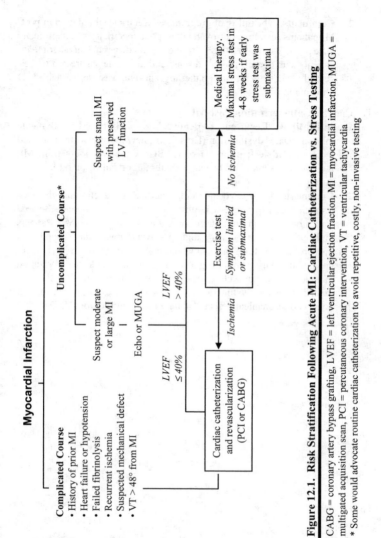

Figure 12.1. Risk Stratification Following Acute MI: Cardiac Catheterization vs. Stress Testing

CABG = coronary artery bypass grafting, LVEF = left ventricular ejection fraction, MI = myocardial infarction, MUGA = multigated acquisition scan, PCI = percutaneous coronary intervention, VT = ventricular tachycardia
* Some would advocate routine cardiac catheterization to avoid repetitive, costly, non-invasive testing

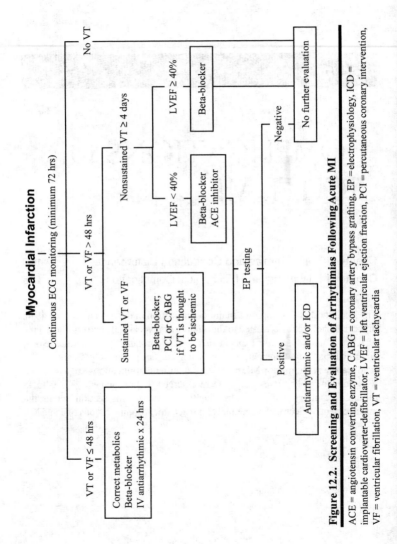

Figure 12.2. Screening and Evaluation of Arrhythmias Following Acute MI

ACE = angiotensin converting enzyme, CABG = coronary artery bypass grafting, EP = electrophysiology, ICD = implantable cardioverter-defibrillator, LVEF = left ventricular ejection fraction, PCI = percutaneous coronary intervention, VF = ventricular fibrillation, VT = ventricular tachycardia

COMPLICATIONS OF ACUTE MI

Chapter 13. Arrhythmias and Conduction Disturbances 109

Chapter 14. Ischemic and Mechanical Complications 125

The likelihood of developing a major complication in the days following acute myocardial infarction is related to the amount of myocardial necrosis, the degree of LV dysfunction, and the extent of residual coronary artery disease. Some complications are transient, easily managed, and relatively benign (e.g., bradycardia with inferior MI, pericarditis); other complications are associated with high mortality rates and require emergency management (e.g., shock, ruptured papillary muscle, ventricular tachycardia). This section details the management of electrical, ischemic, and mechanical complications of acute MI.

Chapter 13

Arrhythmias and Conduction Disturbances in Acute Myocardial Infarction

Sinus Tachycardia

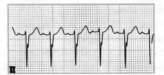

A. **Overview.** There are many potential causes of sinus tachycardia in the setting of ACS, including myocardial ischemia or infarction, heart failure, drug-induced (e.g., dobutamine, dopamine, vasodilators), pericarditis, atrial infarction, acute mitral regurgitation, and VSD. Sinus tachycardia can also be a physiological response to pain, anxiety, fever, hypovolemia, hypoxemia, or hypotension. Sinus tachycardia is associated with larger infarctions and increased mortality risk.[233]

B. **ECG Characteristics.** Sinus P waves at a rate > 100 per minute. P wave amplitude often increases and the PR interval often shortens with increasing heart rates.[6]

C. **Treatment.** Directed at the underlying cause (e.g., myocardial ischemia, pain, anxiety, hypovolemia, fever, heart failure). Drug therapy should not be used to slow reflex tachycardia caused by hypovolemia or compensatory tachycardia caused by heart failure.

Sinus Bradycardia

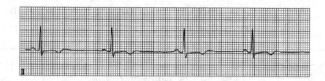

A. Overview.[234-237] Sinus bradycardia occurs in up to one-third of patients with acute MI and is more common with inferior MI and following coronary reperfusion. In the setting of ACS, common causes include high vagal tone (Bezold-Jarisch reflex with inferior MI) and drugs (beta-blockers, verapamil, diltiazem, digitalis, Type IA/IB/IC antiarrhythmics, amiodarone, sotalol). Sinus bradycardia often occurs in conjunction with sinus arrest, sinoatrial exit block, AV junctional escape rhythm, and bradycardia alternating with tachycardia as a component of the Sick Sinus Syndrome.

B. ECG Characteristics. Sinus P waves at a rate < 60 per minute.[6]

C. Treatment. No treatment is indicated for asymptomatic patients. Atropine should be considered for heart rates < 50-60 bpm with associated hypotension, ischemia, or ventricular arrhythmias, at a dose of 0.5-1.0 mg IV; this may be repeated up to a total dose of 3 mg. (Atropine can cause paradoxical slowing of heart rate at low [< 0.5 mg] doses and myocardial ischemia at high doses.) Transcutaneous or transvenous pacing is indicated for symptomatic bradycardia unresponsive to atropine. Dopamine 5-20 mcg/kg/min IV or epinephrine 2-10 mcg/min IV can be used for refractory cases.

Sinus Pause/Arrest

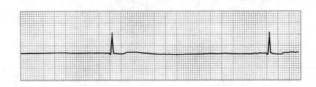

A. **Overview**. Sinus pauses and sinus arrest are due to transient failure of impulse formation at the sinoatrial (SA) node. They occur infrequently with acute MI but are more common with inferior MI and following coronary reperfusion.

B. **ECG Characteristics.** PP interval (pause) exceeds 1.6-2.0 seconds and is not a multiple of the basic sinus PP interval. Sinus pauses must be differentiated from sinus arrhythmia (phasic, gradual change in PP interval); Mobitz Type I second-degree sinoatrial exit block (progressive shortening of the PP interval until a P wave fails to appear); Mobitz Type II second-degree sinoatrial block (PP pause is a multiple of the basic sinus PP interval); abrupt change in autonomic tone (e.g., vagal reaction); and "pseudo" sinus pauses from nonconducted atrial premature complexes (P wave appears to be absent but is actually buried in the T wave, as suggested by subtle deformity of the T wave at the beginning of the pause). Complete failure of sinoatrial conduction (third-degree sinoatrial exit block) cannot be differentiated from complete sinus arrest on surface ECG.[6]

C. **Treatment.** Sinus pauses > 3 seconds and frequent sinus pauses associated with hypotension, heart failure, or other low output symptoms should be treated the same as symptomatic sinus bradycardia (p. 110).

Atrial Flutter

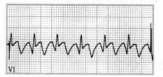

A. Overview.[238,239] Atrial flutter is an uncommon arrhythmia during ACS and suggests associated atrial disease.

B. ECG Characteristics. Rapid, regular, atrial undulations (flutter or "F" waves) usually at a rate of 240-340 per minute. Typical atrial flutter morphology is usually present, with inverted F waves without an isoelectric baseline ("picket-fence" or "sawtooth" appearance) in leads II, III and aVF, and small, positive deflections with a distinct isoelectric baseline in lead V_1. QRS complexes are usually normal but can be wide in the setting of underlying bundle branch block or aberrancy. The AV conduction ratio (ratio of flutter waves to QRS complexes) is usually a fixed, even number (e.g., 2:1, 4:1), but AV conduction can be variable (e.g., 2:1 and 4:1 in the same tracing). Odd-numbered conduction ratios (1:1, 3:1) are uncommon. Atrial flutter with 1:1 AV conduction often conducts aberrantly, resulting in a wide QRS tachycardia that may be confused for VT. In untreated patients, conduction ratios ≥ 4:1 suggest the presence of AV conduction system disease. Carotid sinus massage can unmask flutter waves and help confirm the diagnosis of atrial flutter with 2:1 AV block but does not convert the arrhythmia; discontinuation of carotid sinus massage usually results in return to the original ventricular rate. Flutter rate may be slower (200-240 per minute) in the presence of Type IA, IC, III antiarrhythmic drugs or massively dilated atria, and atypical atrial flutter can exhibit upright F waves in the inferior leads.[6]

C. Treatment. Cardioversion is required if there is associated hemodynamic compromise. Ibutilide should be avoided in ACS due to the increased risk of torsade de pointes. IV and oral amiodarone can be used to maintain sinus rhythm if atrial flutter recurs after cardioversion. Beta-blockers are recommended for rate control in persistent atrial flutter. Anticoagulation should be considered for 3 weeks prior to attempted cardioversion for atrial flutter > 48 hours in duration unless the patient is already receiving IV anticoagulation.

Atrial Fibrillation

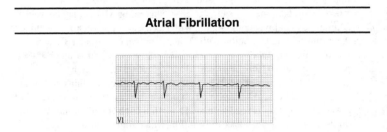

A. **Overview.**[240-244,248,248a] Atrial fibrillation (AF) occurs in 10-15% of patients with acute MI. Risk factors include age > 70 years, acidosis, hypoxemia, hypokalemia, hypomagnesemia, large anterior MI, or MI complicated by heart failure, pericarditis, atrial infarction, or acute mitral regurgitation with left atrial distension. AF often occurs within the first 24 hours of symptom onset, and episodes are frequently transient but may recur. The incidence of systemic embolization is 2% in paroxysmal AF and < 1% in sustained AF. Most embolic events occur by day 4 and 50% occur within the first 24 hours. AF portends a worse prognosis in acute MI.

B. **ECG Characteristics.** P waves are absent, and atrial activity, which is best seen in leads V_1, V_2, II, III and aVF, is totally irregular and represented by fibrillatory (f) waves of varying amplitude, duration, and morphology, which cause random oscillation of the baseline. The ventricular rhythm is irregularly irregular in most cases but can be regular in the presence of complete heart block (e.g., digitalis toxicity). Ventricular rates are 100-180 per minute in the absence of AV nodal blocking agents. Ventricular rates < 100 per minute suggest coexistent AV conduction system disease; rates > 200-220 per minute suggest the presence of an accessory pathway.[6]

C. **Treatment.** No treatment is required for brief, well-tolerated episodes. Immediate DC cardioversion is required for AF resulting in ischemia, hypotension, or heart failure. Stable patients with persistent AF can be managed by rate control with a beta-blocker, diltiazem, digoxin, or amiodarone (especially for patients with heart failure of LV dysfunction), followed by electrical or chemical cardioversion. Sotalol or dofetilide can be used for chemical conversion of AF in patients with preserved LV function; dofetilide is recommended for patients with LV dysfunction (EF < 0.40). Amiodarone is not effective for converting AF but may be used as adjunctive therapy in combination with electrical cardioversion. Sustained AF requires anticoagulation with IV heparin to maintain the PTT at 50-70 seconds. Recent data from the AFFIRM study showed that among 4060 patients with atrial fibrillation and a high risk of stroke or death, rate control plus anticoagulation resulted in a trend toward lower mortality at 5 years (21.3% vs. 23.8%, p = 0.08) and significantly less rehospitalization and fewer adverse drug reactions than did rhythm control with antiarrhythmic drugs. For AF > 48 hours in duration when sinus rhythm is preferred, warfarin is recommended for 3 weeks prior to attempted cardioversion, unless transesophageal echocardiography (TEE) confirms the absence of LV or atrial clot. With or without TEE, anticoagulation is required during and for a minimum of 4 weeks after cardioversion. Correction of acidosis, hypoxemia, and electrolyte disturbances is mandatory for all patients.

Accelerated Idioventricular Rhythm

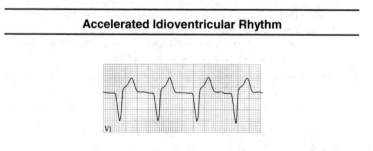

A. Overview.[245-247] Accelerated idioventricular rhythm (AIVR) is not associated with an increased risk of VF or late mortality. In the setting of ACS, common causes include myocardial ischemia and coronary reperfusion. AIVR can also be caused by digitalis toxicity.

B. ECG Characteristics. Regular or slightly irregular ventricular rhythm at a rate of 60-110 per minute. QRS morphology is similar to VPCs. AV dissociation, ventricular capture complexes, and fusion beats are common because of the competition between normal sinus and ectopic ventricular rhythms.[6]

C. Treatment. No treatment is usually necessary, and prophylaxis against VF is not recommended.

Ventricular Tachycardia

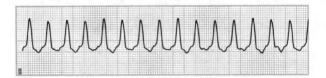

A. Overview.[248,249] Most episodes of ventricular tachycardia (VT) associated with acute MI occur within the first 48 hours of symptom onset. In contrast to early VT, which has no impact on prognosis after hospital discharge, VT after 48 hours increases the risk of late mortality and is an indication for cardiac catheterization. Nonsustained VT occurs in two-thirds of patients within the first 12 hours of MI and does not increase mortality risk. VT can also be induced by electrolyte disturbances (hypokalemia, hyperkalemia, hypomagnesemia), hypoxemia, acidosis, drug toxicity (e.g., digitalis), and LV aneurysm.

B. ECG Characteristics. Rapid succession of 3 or more ventricular premature complexes at a rate > 100 per minute. Nonsustained VT lasts < 30 seconds; sustained VT lasts > 30 seconds or requires intervention due to hemodynamic instability. The RR interval is usually regular but can be irregular. AV dissociation is common, and retrograde atrial activation, fusion complexes, and ventricular capture complexes are occasionally seen. Rarely, VT can present as a narrow QRS tachycardia.[6]

C. Treatment. For well-tolerated VT (i.e., no hypotension or ischemic symptoms) at a rate < 150 per minute, drug therapy can be attempted prior to cardioversion. Procainamide, sotalol, amiodarone, or lidocaine is recommended for patients with normal LV function, and amiodarone or lidocaine is recommended for patients with poor LV function. Poorly-tolerated monomorphic VT requires immediate synchronized cardioversion. Rapid, polymorphic VT should be treated the same as ventricular fibrillation (see below). Correction of acidosis, hypoxemia, electrolyte disturbances, and ongoing ischemia is mandatory for all patients.

Ventricular Fibrillation

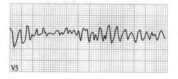

A. **Overview.**[248,250-256] Primary ventricular fibrillation (VF) occurs within the first 4 hours of MI in 4% of patients and is a major cause of early mortality, but early VF does not increase the risk of death after hospital discharge. Prophylaxis with lidocaine or beta-blockers reduces the incidence of primary VF, but routine lidocaine prophylaxis is not recommended due to the risk of increased overall mortality from asystole and other serious bradyarrhythmias. VF can usually be converted into a more stable rhythm when defibrillation occurs within the first minute, but defibrillation is successful in < 25% of cases when initiated after 4 minutes.

B. **ECG Characteristics.** VF is an extremely rapid and irregular ventricular rhythm with chaotic, irregular deflections of varying amplitude and contour and the lack of distinct P waves, QRS complexes, or T waves.[6]

C. **Treatment.** VF requires ACLS and immediately defibrillation up to 3 times. Epinephrine 1 mg IV push every 3-5 minutes or vasopressin 40 U IV push one time only should be administered for persistent VF, followed within 30-60 seconds by repeat defibrillation. Amiodarone or lidocaine should be considered for refractory VF, and magnesium (1-2 gm IV) may be useful for torsades de pointes or hypomagnesemia. Procainamide is an option for intermittent or recurrent VF but is not recommended acutely due to its long administration time. Serum K^+ and Mg^{++} levels should be maintained above 4.0 mEq/L and 2.0 mEq/L, respectively, and acidosis, hypoxemia, ongoing ischemia, and heart failure must be treated aggressively. Routine prophylactic lidocaine has been associated with a trend toward increased mortality and is not recommended.[257]

AV Block, 1°

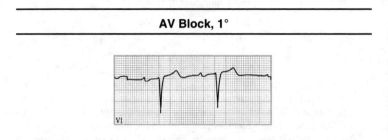

A. **Overview.** 1° AV block is more common with inferior MI, due to associated high vagal tone. It can also be drug-induced (e.g., digitalis, quinidine, procainamide, flecainide, propafenone, amiodarone, sotalol, beta-blockers, diltiazem, verapamil) and can occur in normal individuals.

B. **ECG Characteristics.** PR interval > 0.20 seconds, and each P wave is followed by a QRS complex. The PR interval is usually 0.21-0.40 seconds but can be up to 0.80 seconds in duration. A prolonged PR interval with a narrow QRS complex identifies the site of block in the AV node. If the QRS is wide, conduction delay or block is usually in the His-Purkinje system, although block in the AV node with underlying bundle branch block or aberrancy can present in a similar fashion.[6]

C. **Treatment.** No treatment is usually required. Rare patients with very long (> 0.40 sec) PR intervals and symptoms of low cardiac output may benefit from AV sequential pacing.

AV Block, 2° - Mobitz Type I (Wenckebach)

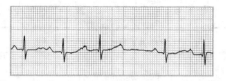

A. **Overview.** In the setting of ACS, common causes include myocardial infarction (especially inferior MI) and drugs (digitalis, beta-blockers, non-dihydropyridine calcium antagonists, flecainide, sotalol, amiodarone, propafenone). Type I block is generally benign and usually occurs at the level of the AV node, resulting in a narrow QRS complex. (In contrast, Mobitz Type II block usually occurs within or below the bundle of His, resulting in a wide QRS complex in 80%, and requires pacing.) Type I block can also occur in normal individuals.

B. **ECG Characteristics.** Progressive lengthening of the PR interval and progressive shortening of the RR interval until a P wave is blocked, and the RR interval containing the nonconducted P wave is less than 2 PP intervals. Classical Wenckebach periodicity is not always evident, especially when sinus arrhythmia is present or an abrupt change in autonomic tone occurs (e.g., vagal reaction). In Type I block with high conduction ratios (i.e., infrequent pauses), the PR interval of the beats immediately preceding the blocked P wave may be equal to each other, suggesting Type II block. In these situations, it is best to compare the PR interval immediately before and after the blocked P wave: a difference in the PR interval suggests Type I block, whereas a constant PR interval suggests Type II block. Mobitz Type I 2° AV block results in "group" or "pattern beating" due to the presence of nonconducted P waves. Other causes of group beating include blocked APCs, Type II second-degree AV block, and concealed His-bundle depolarizations.[6]

C. **Treatment.** No treatment is indicated for asymptomatic patients. Atropine (0.5-2.0 mg) followed by pacing can be used to treat symptomatic patients with frequent nonconducted beats and associated hypotension, heart failure, or other low output symptoms. Aminophylline may be of value in the setting of myocardial ischemia to reduce high tissue adenosine levels, which can impair AV conduction.

AV Block, 2° - Mobitz Type II

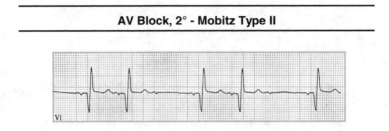

A. **Overview.** Mobitz Type II block is almost always due to serious conduction system disease and is associated with an increased risk of progression to complete heart block.

B. **ECG Characteristics.** Regular sinus or atrial rhythm with intermittent nonconducted P waves and no evidence for atrial prematurity. The PR interval in the conducted beats is constant, and the RR interval containing the nonconducted P wave is equal to 2 PP intervals. Type II block may be confused for Type I block with high conduction rates (e.g., 10:9 conduction). In these situations, it is best to compare the PR interval immediately before and after the blocked P wave: a difference in the PR interval suggests Type I block, whereas a constant PR interval suggests Type II block.[6]

C. **Treatment.** Temporary followed by permanent pacing is indicated for Mobitz Type II block, regardless of symptomatic status.

AV Block, 3° (Complete Heart Block)

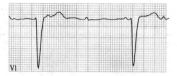

A. Overview.[258-261] Complete heart block occurs in 5-15% of patients with acute MI. In inferior MI, complete heart block is usually preceded by first-degree AV block and typically occurs at the level of the AV node. In these cases, heart block is often associated with a stable junctional escape rhythm (narrow QRS complex at a rate > 40 per minute) and usually lasts < 1 week. In anterior MI, complete heart block occurs as a result of extensive damage to the left ventricle and is often preceded by Type II second-degree AV block or bifascicular block. Mortality rates are very high (up to 70%), due to pump failure rather than heart block, per se.

B. ECG Characteristics. Atrial impulses consistently fail to reach the ventricles, resulting in independent atrial and ventricular rhythms. This manifests as a varying PR interval with constant PP and RR intervals. The P wave may precede, be buried in, or follow the QRS. Ventricular rhythm is maintained by a junctional or idioventricular escape rhythm or a ventricular pacemaker. Ventriculophasic sinus arrhythmia (i.e., PP interval containing a QRS complex is shorter than the PP interval without a QRS complex) occurs in 30-50%.[6]

C. Treatment. The site and stability of the escape rhythm determines the need and urgency for intervention. No treatment is usually necessary for stable patients with narrow escape complexes. For symptomatic patients and those with wide-complex escape rhythms, temporary pacing is indicated. Permanent pacing is usually required for persistent heart block > 5 days and for complete heart block that is preceded by Mobitz Type II second-degree AV block or accompanied by bundle branch block. It is important to exclude reversible causes of complete heart block, including digitalis toxicity and hyperkalemia.

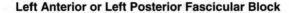

Left Anterior or Left Posterior Fascicular Block

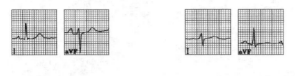

LAFB   *LPFB*

A. **Overview.**[262,264] Compared to the left anterior fascicle, the left posterior fascicle is shorter and thicker and receives dual blood supply from both the left and right coronary arteries. In acute MI, the incidence of isolated left anterior fascicular block (LAFB) and isolated left posterior fascicular block (LPFB) is 4% and 0.4%, respectively. LAFB usually occurs in the setting of anteroseptal or anterolateral infarction, and the LAD is typically the infarct vessel. When LPFB develops during acute MI, multivessel disease with extensive infarction is usually present and the prognosis is poor.

B. **ECG Characteristics.** <u>LAFB</u>: Left axis deviation with mean QRS axis between −45 and −90 degrees; qR complex (or an R wave) in leads I and aVL; rS complex in lead III; normal or slightly prolonged QRS duration (0.08-0.10 seconds); and no other factors responsible for left axis deviation (e.g., LVH, inferior MI, chronic lung disease, left bundle branch block, ostium premium atrial septal defect, severe hyperkalemia). <u>LPFB</u>: Right axis deviation with mean QRS axis between 100 and 180 degrees; normal or slightly prolonged QRS duration (0.08-0.10 seconds); rS complex in leads I and VL; qR complex in lead III; and no other factors responsible for right axis deviation (e.g., RVH, vertical heart, chronic lung disease, pulmonary embolism, lateral MI, dextrocardia, lead reversal, Wolff-Parkinson-White syndrome).[6]

C. **Treatment.** No treatment is required for isolated hemiblock. Pacing may be indicated when LAFB or LPFB is accompanied by right bundle branch block (see bifascicular block, p. 124).

Right Bundle Branch Block (RBBB)

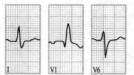

A. **Overview.**[264-267] Complete RBBB occurs in 5% of patients with acute (usually anterior) MI, often in conjunction with left anterior fascicular block. RBBB is associated with an increased risk of death post-MI. Normal adults with RBBB (incidence 0.2%) have essentially the same prognosis as the general population.

B. **ECG Characteristics.** Prolonged QRS duration ($\geq$ 0.12 seconds); secondary R wave (R') in leads V_1 and V_2 (rsR' or rSR'), with R' usually taller than the initial R wave; delayed onset of intrinsicoid deflection (beginning of QRS complex to peak of R wave > 0.05 seconds) and secondary ST-T changes (T wave inversion $\pm$ downsloping ST segments) in leads V_1 and V_2; and wide, slurred S waves in leads I, V_5, and V_6. In RBBB, the mean QRS axis is determined by the initial unblocked 0.06-0.08 seconds of the QRS and should be normal unless left anterior fascicular block or left posterior fascicular block is present. RBBB does not interfere with the ability to detect ventricular hypertrophy or Q-waves on ECG.[6]

C. **Treatment.** No treatment is indicated for isolated RBBB. Transcutaneous pacing patches (or possibly temporary transvenous pacing) can be considered for RBBB accompanied by first-degree AV block.

Left Bundle Branch Block (LBBB)

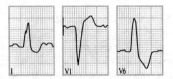

A. **Overview.**[7,263,268,269] LBBB occurs in 1-2% of patients with acute (usually anterior) MI and is associated with an increased risk of complete heart block and death. In-hospital mortality rates up to 25% have been reported.

B. **ECG Characteristics.** Prolonged QRS duration (≥ 0.12 seconds); delayed onset of intrinsicoid deflection (beginning of QRS to peak of R wave > 0.05 seconds) in leads V_5 and V_6; broad monophasic R waves in leads I, V_5, and V_6, which are usually notched or slurred; secondary ST-T changes opposite in direction to the major QRS deflection (i.e., ST depression and T wave inversion in leads I, V_5, and V_6; ST elevation and upright T waves in leads V_1 and V_2); and rS or QS complexes in the right precordial leads. Left axis deviation may be present. LBBB interferes with the ability to detect QRS axis, ventricular hypertrophy, and acute MI on ECG.[6]

C. **Treatment.** Transcutaneous pacing patches (or possibly temporary transvenous pacing) is indicated for isolated LBBB. For LBBB with first-degree AV block, temporary transvenous pacing is recommended.

Bifascicular Block or
Alternating Bundle Branch Block

A. **Overview and ECG Characteristics.** RBBB with LAFB occurs in 5% of patients with acute (usually anterior) MI, and the usual infarct vessel is the LAD. RBBB with LPFB is uncommon in acute MI (incidence < 1%) and indicates the presence of multivessel disease. Alternating bundle branch block is associated with an increased risk of progression to complete heart block and can present as RBBB alternating with LBBB or as RBBB with alternating LAFB and LPFB.[6]

B. **Treatment.** Temporary transvenous pacing is recommended for alternating bundle branch block of any age and for new or indeterminate age bifascicular block with first-degree AV block. Permanent pacing is indicated for bifascicular or alternating bundle branch block associated with complete heart block or second-degree AV block in the His-Purkinje system, regardless of symptoms.

Chapter 14

Ischemic and Mechanical Complications

Failed Fibrinolysis (Chapter 5)

A. **Overview.** Only 55% of vessels achieve TIMI-3 flow after fibrinolytic therapy, and there are no clinical markers to accurately predict reperfusion. In small randomized trials, rescue PCI improved regional wall motion and LV function after failed fibrinolysis and reduced the risk of recurrent ischemia, heart failure, shock, and death in high-risk patients. However, early mortality was high (> 30%) if rescue PTCA failed. In GUSTO-III, use of abciximab during rescue PTCA reduced mortality rates at 30 days.

B. **Treatment.** Emergency angiography should be considered for ongoing chest pain, hemodynamic instability, or persistent ST-elevation 90 minutes after lytic therapy, especially for large anterior MI. Stents plus GP IIb/IIIa inhibitors are recommended for high-grade lesions with impaired coronary flow.

Left Ventricular Aneurysm

A. **Overview.**[270-274] LV aneurysm develops in up to 10% of acute (usually anterior) infarctions, typically within the first 3 months. Important risk factors include a persistently occluded vessel and poor collateral blood flow. Early reperfusion therapy and ACE inhibitors reduce infarct expansion and LV aneurysm formation.

B. **Diagnosis.** A thinned, smooth, dyskinetic ventricular wall is evident on echocardiogram or ventriculogram. Persistent ST-elevation in the region of the aneurysm is often present on ECG.

C. **Complications.** LV aneurysms predispose to heart failure, mitral regurgitation, late ventricular arrhythmias, and sudden death. Mural thrombus is common on autopsy, and systemic thromboembolism occurs in

2-5%. The risk of cardiac rupture is much greater with pseudoaneurysm (see below) than with true aneurysm.

D. Treatment. Surgical resection is indicated for aneurysms causing heart failure, angina, systemic thromboembolism, or recurrent VT/VF. Aneurysmectomy often improves ejection fraction and functional status, and resection is usually combined with CABG ± EP-mapping of arrhythmias. Associated papillary muscle dysfunction may require mitral valve repair or replacement, and inducibility of VT may require ICD implantation. Operative mortality is 10%.

Left Ventricular Pseudoaneurysm

A. Overview.[273-276] Pseudoaneurysms are contained free-wall ruptures protected from exsanguinating hemorrhage by clot in the pericardial space. In contrast to the walls of true aneurysms, which are composed of endocardial tissue and fibrosed myocardium, pseudoaneurysmal walls are composed only of pericardium and thrombus, increasing the risk of cardiac rupture. Pseudoaneurysms usually involve the anterior-apical or infero-posterior walls of the left ventricle.

B. Diagnosis. Narrow neck opening into the body of the pseudoaneurysm is evident on echocardiogram or ventriculogram.

C. Treatment. Prompt surgical resection is usually recommended, even in clinically stable patients, due to the increased risk of cardiac rupture and death.

Left Ventricular Dysfunction (Acute Heart Failure)

A. Overview.[277,278] In the setting of acute MI, acute heart failure is often a result of both systolic and diastolic LV dysfunction (i.e., decreased contractility and compliance). Other causes of low output failure include RV infarction, mechanical defects (e.g., acute MR, VSD), bradyarrhythmias (e.g., sinus arrest, AV junctional rhythm), tachyarrhythmias (e.g., atrial fibrillation, SVT, VT), and conduction disturbances (e.g., high-degree AV block). Recovery of diastolic and systolic function can be delayed for days or weeks after successful coronary reperfusion due to stunned myocardium.

B. Presentation. Depending on the extent of LV dysfunction, symptoms can vary from mild pulmonary congestion to acute pulmonary edema to severe low cardiac output with cardiogenic shock.

C. Treatment (Figure 14.1). The immediate goals of therapy are to treat reversible factors, control symptoms, and maintain vital organ perfusion. Patients with normal blood pressure should be treated acutely with furosemide, sublingual or spray nitroglycerin, and morphine. Dobutamine (and/or milrinone) and IV nitroglycerin are added for persistent symptoms, and nitroprusside is added for severe hypertension or acute mitral regurgitation. Patients with hypotension should be treated with dopamine, followed by IABP counterpulsation ± norepinephrine for persistent hypotension. Endotracheal intubation with mechanical ventilation may be required to maintain oxygenation, prevent CO_2 retention, redistribute blood flow out of the pulmonary circuit, and decrease the work of breathing. Proper management also requires treatment of ongoing ischemia, mechanical defects, arrhythmias, and conduction disturbances. Once patients have been stabilized on IV medications x 48-72 hours, they can usually be switched to oral therapy. ACE inhibitors and beta-blockers improve long-term outcome.

D. Prognosis. In-hospital mortality ranges from 5% for patients with normal LV function to 50-80% for patients with cardiogenic shock.

Left Ventricular Thrombus

A. Overview.[279-281] LV thrombus develops in up to 20% of patients with acute (usually anterior) MI, typically within the first 5 days. Most embolic events occur in the first 3 months, and the risk of embolism is increased for mobile or protruding thrombi.

B. Treatment. Consider IV heparin during hospitalization followed by warfarin (INR 2.0-3.0) x 3 months, especially for mobile or protruding LV thrombi associated with anterior MI, to reduce the risk of embolization (Cardiovasc Rev Rep 1986;7:183). Randomized trials are underway to examine the preferred mode of antithrombotic therapy in these patients.

Acute Heart Failure[1]

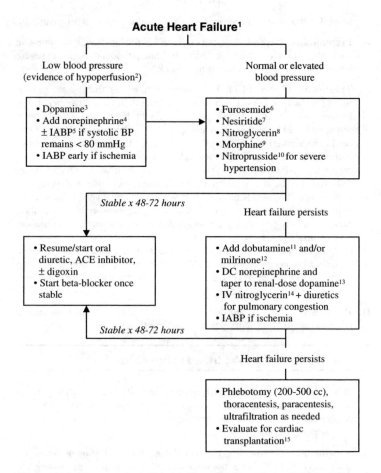

Figure 14.1. Management of Acute Heart Failure Secondary to ACS

See footnotes, next page.

Footnotes for Figure 14.1.

ACE = angiotensin converting enzyme, BP = blood pressure, DC = discontinue, IABP = intra-aortic ballon pump, PA = pulmonary artery

1. Assess airway, breathing circulation; administer oxygen; start IV; intubate early for severe respiratory distress, acidosis, hypotension; pulse oximeter, blood pressure cuff, ECG monitor; obtain 12-lead ECG and treat arrhythmias and heart block; obtain CBC, electrolytes, portable chest x-ray, and echocardiogram when feasible; utilize arterial line for hypotension and pulmonary artery catheter when feasible; treat reversible causes and precipitating factors (e.g., ongoing ischemia, ventricular septal defect, papillary muscle rupture).
2. Cool clammy skin, impaired cognition, oliguria, azotemia.
3. Dopamine 5-20 mcg/kg/min IV infusion.
4. Norepinephrine 0.5-20 mcg/min IV infusion.
5. Intra-aortic balloon counterpulsation is contraindicated in the presence of moderate-to-severe aortic regurgitation.
6. Furosemide 0.5-1.0 mg/kg IV. Up to 100-200 mg IV may be needed for patients receiving long-term diuretic therapy.
7. Nesiritide 2 mcg/kg IV bolus followed by an IV infusion of 0.01 mcg/kg/min.
8. Nitroglycerin 0.4 mg SL or spray every 5 minutes.
9. Morphine 1-5 mg IV over 1-5 minutes; may repeat dose every 5-30 minutes x 3.
10. Nitroprusside 0.1-5.0 mcg/kg/min IV infusion.
11. Dobutamine 2-30 mcg/kg/min IV infusion.
12. Milrinone 50 mcg/kg IV bolus over 10 minutes plus 0.375-0.75 mcg/kg/min IV infusion.
13. Renal dose dopamine 2 mcg/kg/min IV infusion.
14. IV nitroglycerin 10-100 mcg/min IV infusion. Tachyphylaxis can occur as early as 24 hours after continuous IV therapy.
15. IABP or ventricular assist device may be needed as a bridge to cardiac transplantation.

Mitral Regurgitation: *Ruptured Papillary Muscle/Chordae*

A. **Overview.**[282-285] Papillary muscle rupture complicates 1% of acute (usually inferior) infarctions caused by right coronary artery (most common) or left circumflex coronary artery occlusion. The posteromedial papillary muscle has a single blood supply from the posterior descending branch of the dominant coronary artery and is more likely to rupture than the anterolateral papillary muscle, which receives a dual blood supply from the left anterior descending and left circumflex coronary arteries.

B. **Presentation.** Papillary muscle rupture or ruptured chordae should be suspected in patients who develop acute pulmonary edema 2-9 days post-MI. (Rupture is less common within the first 24 hours.) A new apical systolic mitral regurgitation murmur may or may not be present, and the infarct can be large or small.

C. **Diagnosis.** Transthoracic or transesophageal echocardiography with Doppler imaging is used to confirm the diagnosis of ruptured papillary muscle and exclude other mechanical defects (e.g., VSD, LV aneurysm or pseudoaneurysm, free wall rupture). Echocardiography demonstrates a flail or prolapsing mitral valve leaflet with regurgitant jet flow into the left atrium, although the severity of acute MR is often underestimated by echo. A prominent V-wave is frequently seen in the pulmonary capillary wedge pressure tracing.

D. **Treatment.** Emergency surgical repair is recommended, even in hemodynamically stable patients, due to the risk of acute decompensation. Stabilizing measures prior to surgery include IABP counterpulsation, sodium nitroprusside, and possibly inotropes.

E. **Prognosis.** Mortality rates are high with medical treatment (70-90%) or surgery (20-50%).

Mitral Regurgitation: *Ischemic Papillary Muscle*

A. **Overview.** Ischemic papillary muscle dysfunction is more common after inferior MI, usually involves the posteromedial papillary muscle, and can occur in large or small infarcts.

B. Presentation. Transient papillary muscle dysfunction can cause acute (flash) pulmonary edema in otherwise stable patients. An apical systolic murmur can be persistent, intermittent, or absent.

C. Diagnosis. Echocardiogram demonstrates mitral regurgitation, which can be persistent or transient (due to intermittent ischemia). A prolapsing mitral valve may or may not be present. A prominent V-wave is sometimes seen in the pulmonary capillary wedge pressure tracing during episodes of flash pulmonary edema.

D. Treatment. Vasodilators should be used to stabilize the patient; if unsuccessful, IABP counterpulsation is often effective. Revascularization with PCI[285a] or CABG[285b] should be considered.

Acute Pericarditis

A. Overview.[286-291] Acute pericarditis complicates 10-15% of acute infarctions, usually 2-4 days following Q-wave (transmural) MI. Persistent or recurrent chest pain within the first 24 hours of acute MI is unlikely to be caused by pericarditis.

B. Presentation. The most common symptom is pleuritic-type chest pain, which radiates to left trapezial ridge and is relieved by sitting forward. ECG findings include J-point elevation, PR-segment depression, and concave upward ST-segment elevation, which can be diffuse but is more often localized to the area of transmural necrosis. A 3-component pericardial friction rub may be present, but the absence of a friction rub does not exclude acute pericarditis. Pericardial effusion occurs in 40%, but cardiac tamponade is infrequent, and a small pericardial effusion can accompany acute MI in absence of pericarditis. Pericarditis does not cause an elevation in cardiac markers.

C. Treatment. Aspirin 160-325 mg PO q24h is recommended, and doses up to 650 mg PO q4-6h may be required. Refractory cases often benefit from indomethacin ± corticosteroids (e.g., prednisone 60-80 mg/d x 5-7 days, then discontinued gradually), but these agents should be used sparingly since they can increase coronary vascular resistance, impair infarct healing,[292] and possibly increase the risk of myocardial rupture.[293] Pericarditis is a relative contraindication for anticoagulation and a strong contraindication for fibrinolytic therapy. All patients with pericarditis require close monitoring for enlarging pericardial effusion and impending cardiac tamponade.

Pericarditis, Dressler's Syndrome

A. **Overview.**[294-296] Dressler's syndrome is an immunologic reaction that presents as a pleuropericarditis 1-12 weeks after acute MI in 1-3% of patients. It is generally benign and self-limited, but recurrences are common and constrictive pericarditis can occur.

B. **Presentation.** Symptoms include fever, chest pain, pericardial and pleural effusions. ECG findings are typical of pericarditis, with diffuse, concave upward ST-segment elevation.

C. **Treatment.** Treated the same as acute pericarditis post-MI (p. 131).

Recurrent Ischemia

A. **Overview.** Post-infarct angina is more common after fibrinolysis (30%) than after primary PCI (10%) and is associated with an increased risk of reinfarction and death. In the DANAMI trial of revascularization vs. medical therapy for spontaneous or inducible ischemia after fibrinolysis, revascularization reduced reinfarction, unstable angina, and the need for antianginal medications at 12-24 months.[112]

B. **Treatment.** Recommendations include resumption of IV heparin or SQ enoxaparin (for rest angina), continuation of beta-blockers and nitrates, and triage to cardiac catheterization and revascularization (PCI/CABG).

Reinfarction

A. **Overview.**[297-300] Reinfarction is more common after fibrinolytic therapy (4%) than after medical therapy or PCI for ST-elevation MI (< 1-2%). It also is more common after non-Q-wave MI than after Q-wave MI. Reinfarction is associated with further reductions in ejection fraction and an increased risk of cardiogenic shock and death. The risk of reinfarction is reduced by aspirin and beta-blockers.

B. **Treatment.** IV heparin or low-molecular-weight heparin, nitroglycerin, morphine sulfate, and triage to catheterization and revascularization (PCI or CABG) are recommended. Fibrinolytic therapy with tPA, rPA, or TNK-tPA can be readministered if the first dose was given ≥ 48 hours earlier, but streptokinase should be avoided within 2 years of previous administration due to the persistence of neutralizing antistreptococcal antibodies.

Right Ventricular Infarction

A. **Overview.**[301-312] RV infarction occurs in 30% of inferior infarcts and 10% of anterior infarcts. Large RV infarcts are complicated by heart block or atrial fibrillation in 20-50%.

B. **Presentation.** Varies from mild, asymptomatic RV dysfunction to cardiogenic shock. Cardiogenic shock can occur with relatively well-preserved LV function.

C. **Diagnosis.** RV infarction is suggested by distended neck veins or Kussmaul's sign (jugular venous distension on inspiration) with or without clear lungs and low blood pressure in the setting of inferior MI. RV infarction should also be suspected when severe hypotension develops after sublingual nitroglycerin. ST-elevation is often present in lead V_1 and right-sided lead V_{4R}, but these findings are transient and resolve within hours in > 50%. Echocardiography demonstrates a hypokinetic, dilated right ventricle with abnormal interventricular and interatrial septal motion. On pulmonary artery catheterization, right atrial pressure exceeds 10 mmHg and the ratio of right atrial pressure to wedge pressure is ≥ 0.8. Right-to-left shunting across a patent foramen ovale should be suspected when arterial oxygen saturation fails to respond to supplemental oxygen.

D. **Treatment.** The most important form of therapy is early reperfusion with PCI or fibrinolysis, which improves RV ejection fraction and reduces the risk of heart block. Other useful measures include maintenance of RV preload with rapid saline infusion (1-2 L), dobutamine (preferred) or dopamine for persistent low cardiac output, AV sequential pacing for high-grade heart block or bradycardia not responding to atropine, cardioversion for hemodynamically-significant SVT or atrial fibrillation, and use of an RV assist device for severe refractory shock. For coexistent LV dysfunction, therapeutic considerations include IABP counterpulsation and careful afterload reduction with ACE inhibitors ± sodium nitroprusside. Nitrates and diuretics can worsen hemodynamics by causing further reductions in preload and should be avoided.

E. Prognosis. RV infarction increases morbidity and mortality associated with inferior MI, even though RV function recovers in most patients within days to weeks. Prognosis is closely related to LV function and residual coronary artery disease.

Cardiac Rupture

A. Overview.[285,313-316] Cardiac free-wall rupture complicates 1-4% of acute infarctions and is the second leading cause of hospital death post-MI. More than 90% of ruptures occur in the first week and up to 40% occur in the first 24 hours. Risk factors include first MI, female gender, advanced age, hypertension, anterior MI, Q-wave MI, persistent chest pain, lack of collateral circulation, no prior angina, use of NSAIDs or corticosteroids, and late (> 12 hours) administration of fibrinolytic therapy. The risk of rupture is reduced by early (< 12 hours) reperfusion and beta-blockers.

B. Presentation. Cardiac rupture presents with recurrent chest pain and acute hemodynamic collapse. Shock, electromechanical dissociation, and cardiac tamponade occur suddenly.

C. Treatment. Immediate surgical repair after rapid confirmation by echocardiography can be lifesaving. Pericardiocentesis should be performed for hypotension or shock en route to emergency surgery.

D. Prognosis. Death is often immediate.

Cardiogenic Shock

A. **Overview.**[317,318] Cardiogenic shock complicates 5-7% of acute infarctions, usually within the first few hours, and is the leading cause of death post-MI. Cardiogenic shock develops when myocardial necrosis exceeds 40% of LV mass, but it may also result from a relatively smaller infarct complicated by hypovolemia, RV infarction, papillary muscle rupture, ventricular septal defect, or cardiac tamponade. Risk factors include large MI, previous MI, admission ejection fraction < 35%, diabetes mellitus, and advanced age. The risk of cardiogenic shock is reduced by early reperfusion.

B. **Presentation.** Persistent hypotension (BP < 90 mmHg) accompanied by hypoperfusion of vital organs, including impaired sensorium, oliguria, and clammy skin. When cardiogenic shock is caused by extensive myocardial necrosis, low cardiac output, elevated systemic vascular resistance and pulmonary capillary wedge pressure, and pulmonary rales are present.

C. **Treatment.** Cardiogenic shock requires aggressive therapy, given the high (70-90%) mortality rates associated with fibrinolytic/medical therapy alone. Immediate angiography, IABP counterpulsation, and revascularization are recommended for patients < 75 years (and possibly for patients > 75 years), based on results from randomized trials and registries (see below). Other measures include IV fluids to optimize filling pressures, dobutamine to enhance cardiac output, dopamine to maintain vital organ perfusion, and treatment of associated mechanical defects, arrhythmias, and conduction disturbances. A left ventricular assist device (LVAD) is sometimes required as a stabilizing bridge to revascularization.

D. **Prognosis.** In GUSTO-I, an aggressive revascularization strategy (PTCA or CABG) was independently associated with improved 30-day survival.[79] In the randomized SHOCK trial comparing emergency revascularization (PTCA or CABG) to initial medical stabilization and later revascularization, 30-day mortality was significantly reduced using the early invasive approach in the following groups: age < 75 years (41% vs. 57%, p < 0.05); randomization within 6 hours of symptom onset (37% vs. 63%, p < 0.01); and prior MI (40% vs. 68%, p < 0.01). Survival benefit persisted at 1 year for patients in the emergency revascularization group (47.6% vs. 33.6%, p < 0.03), and 83% of 1-year survivors were in NYHA heart failure class I or

II.[80] Failure to restore TIMI-3 flow during PCI was associated with higher mortality rates at 30 days (65% vs. 35% if TIMI-3 flow was restored, p < 0.001). Data from the SHOCK trial registry indicated a survival benefit for early revascularization in select patients ≥ 75 years.

Ventricular Septal Defect (VSD)

A. **Overview.**[285,319-324] Acute VSD complicates 0.5-2% of acute infarctions, usually between day 2-5, and is more common after anterior MI than after inferior-posterior MI.

B. **Presentation.** VSD usually presents as a new systolic murmur. Features favoring the diagnosis of VSD over acute mitral regurgitation include a palpable thrill, absence of acute pulmonary edema, lack of a prominent V-wave in the pulmonary capillary wedge pressure tracing, and an oxygen step-up in the high right ventricle. Cardiogenic shock may ensue.

C. **Diagnosis.** VSDs are confirmed by echocardiography with Doppler imaging, which allows visualization of the defect and detection of the shunt. Pulmonary artery catheterization with oximetry reveals a > 5-7% step-up in O_2 saturation of blood between the right atrium and right ventricle.

D. **Treatment.** Early catheterization and surgical intervention are recommended, even in clinically stable patients, despite biased, early surgical series recommending medical stabilization prior to surgical repair. IABP counterpulsation, vasodilators, and inotropes can be used as stabilizing measures during preparation for surgery.

E. **Prognosis.** Mortality rates are high with medical therapy (90%) or surgery (40-60%). Survival is worse for VSDs associated with inferior-posterior MI or RV infarction and for complex septal defects.

Major Depression

A. **Overview.** Major depression occurs in over 15% of patients after acute MI and is an independent risk factor for adverse long-term prognosis. Small studies have demonstrated increased risk of ventricular arrhythmias and death within the first 6 months post-MI, possibly related to altered autonomic tone.[325]

B. **Treatment.** Selective serotonin reuptake inhibitors (SSRI) improve psychosocial functioning and exhibit mild antiplatelet effects post-ACS, but their impact on survival is unknown. Major depression should be distinguished from minor depressive symptoms, which are common after MI and represent a normal adjustment reaction that is often short-lived. Recent data indicate that SSRI treatment after ACS in depressed patients improves depression and may improve clinical outcome.[325a] Cognitive behavior therapy improves depression but does not reduce cardiac events.

Section 6

ACS PITFALLS

Chapter 15
ACS Pitfalls

Pitfall: Delay in diagnosis of ACS

Prompt triage and early therapy improve outcomes in ACS. An abbreviated evaluation including a brief history, physical examination, and ECG should be performed immediately upon arrival, ideally within 10 minutes. The use of emergency department algorithms substantially improves time to diagnosis.

Pitfall: Failure to consider non-ischemic causes of chest pain at patient presentation

Pulmonary embolism, thoracic aorta dissection, and pericarditis can present similarly to ACS and possess ECG and cardiac marker abnormalities. These conditions can progress to life-threatening situations and require expedient diagnosis and treatment.

Pitfall: Failure to recognize acute MI in the absence of chest pain

In the National Registry of Myocardial Infarction 2, one-third of more than 400,000 patients with confirmed MI did not have chest pain on hospital presentation.[326] Women, diabetics, the elderly, and patients with prior heart failure were disproportionately affected. MI patients without chest pain were less likely to be diagnosed on hospital admission (22% vs. 50%); were less likely to receive reperfusion therapy (25% vs. 74%), beta-blockers (28% vs. 48%), or heparin (53% vs. 83%); and were more likely to die in-hospital (23% vs. 9%). Patients with ST-elevation MI presenting with 12 hours of symptom onset should be considered for reperfusion therapy regardless of pain status.

Pitfall: Failure to check serial ECGs in patients with ongoing chest pain but without ST-elevation on initial ECG

Patients presenting with ACS but without ST-elevation on initial ECG occasionally develop complete coronary occlusion and ST-elevation early during their hospital stay. In patients with ongoing or changing ischemic symptoms, serial ECGs should be used to monitor ST-segment shifts. Patients who develop ST-elevation should be considered for reperfusion therapy.

Pitfall: Failure to check a right-sided ECG in inferior MI to identify right ventricular infarction

RV infarction is often associated with inferior MI and can be diagnosed early by documenting ≥ 1 mm ST-elevation in lead V_{4R}. Early recognition of RV infarction can minimize or prevent adverse hemodynamic consequences by alerting clinicians of the need for aggressive intravenous fluid administration and avoidance of nitrates and other vasodilators. The most important form of therapy for RV infarction is early reperfusion therapy, which improves RV ejection fraction and reduces the risk of heart block. Other useful measures include maintenance of RV preload with 1-2 liters of normal saline, dobutamine (preferred) or dopamine for persistent low cardiac output, AV sequential pacing for high-grade heart block or bradycardia unresponsive to atropine, cardioversion for hemodynamically-significant SVT or atrial fibrillation, and use of an RV assist device for refractory shock. Nitrates and diuretics can worsen hemodynamics by further reducing RV preload.

Pitfall: Delay in initiating reperfusion therapy

A number of analyses from randomized clinical trials have demonstrated improved clinical outcomes associated with prompt reperfusion therapy, including smaller infarct size, less ventricular dysfunction, and better survival. For every hour saved in time from symptom onset to treatment, there is an approximate 1% reduction in 30-day mortality. Early symptom recognition and triage are critical components of the overall treatment strategy for ACS. AHA/ACC guidelines have targeted a door-to-needle time within 30 minutes and a door-to-balloon inflation time within 60-120 minutes.[91,92]

Pitfall: Underuse of reperfusion therapy in ST-elevation MI

Reports from the GRACE[25] and NRMI[26] registries indicate that one-third of patients with ST-elevation MI do not receive reperfusion therapy. Common reasons for withholding therapy included advanced age, absence of chest pain, or a history of heart failure, MI, or CABG, none of which is a contraindication to reperfusion therapy. For every 1000 patients treated with fibrinolytic therapy, approximately 20 lives are saved.[7] Furthermore, these benefits are long-lasting: In the 10-year follow-up of the GISSI-I trial,[33] 18 lives were saved for every 1000 patients treated with streptokinase. Similar or greater benefits exist for primary percutaneous coronary intervention. Reperfusion therapy is indicated for all patients with ST-elevation MI < 12 hours.

Pitfall: Underuse of reperfusion therapy in acute MI patients with left bundle branch block (LBBB)

LBBB interferes with the ability to identify ST-elevation MI on ECG. Patients with prolonged ischemic chest pain and new LBBB have high (20-25%) in-hospital mortality rates and derive substantial benefit from fibrinolytic therapy (49 lives saved for every 1000 patients treated).[7] However, patients with LBBB are 78% less likely to receive reperfusion therapy than patients with ST-elevation.[8] Because of their increased risk, patients with new LBBB and symptoms consistent with ACS should receive direct PCI (preferred) or fibrinolytic therapy.

Pitfall: Underuse of reperfusion therapy in elderly patients

Patients over age 75 are 6 times less likely to receive fibrinolytic therapy despite a high risk of death and reinfarction.[73] Although these patients are at increased risk of intracranial hemorrhage when treated with fibrinolytic therapy compared with younger patients, they are also at higher risk of death after MI. Unless specific contraindications exist, patients over age 75 with ST-elevation or new LBBB should undergo direct PCI; if not readily available, the risks and benefits of fibrinolytic therapy should be carefully weighed in this high-risk population.

Pitfall: Inappropriate dosing of heparin, especially in the setting of fibrinolytic therapy

Most current fibrinolytic regimens call for concomitant antithrombin therapy with unfractionated heparin, and judicious dosing of heparin is especially important in this setting. Intravenous heparin dosing and the degree of anticoagulation are directly related to clinical outcomes: The probability of 30-day mortality and reinfarction rises for aPTT values below 50 seconds and above 70 seconds in a classic "J-shaped" therapeutic curve.[328] Higher aPTT values are strongly related to lower patient weight, older age, female gender, and lack of cigarette smoking. These observations have prompted a revision of the AHA/ACC guidelines for heparin dosing in the setting of acute MI. For patients receiving fibrinolytic therapy, intravenous unfractionated heparin is recommended as a 60-70 U/kg IV bolus followed by an IV maintenance infusion of 12-15 U/kg/hr (not to exceed 5000 U bolus and 1000 U/hr infusion), adjusted to aPTT of 1.5-2.5 times control (50-75 seconds).

Pitfall: Misuse of cardiac troponins for risk stratification

Cardiac troponins are more sensitive markers of myocardial injury than CK-MB, but troponins are not generally detectable above the upper limit of normal for 6-8 hours. A single initial negative value does not imply low risk and may, in fact, mask a troponin-positive, high-risk patient. The tendency to minimize the importance of a positive troponin in renal insufficiency is another important and possibly more widespread problem. Troponin values independently predict early outcome and identify patients most likely to benefit from GP IIb/IIIa receptor antagonists and the early invasive approach to management.[15-22]

Pitfall: Not recognizing the high risk associated with non-ST-elevation MI

Compared with ST-elevation MI, non-ST-elevation MI is associated with less myocardial necrosis (smaller infarct), better preservation of LV function, and lower in-hospital mortality. However, since non-ST-elevation infarcts are usually associated with residual viable myocardium supplied by a coronary artery with a high-grade but nonocclusive stenosis, reinfarction rates are higher than after ST-elevation MI. In the GUSTO-IIb study, 1-year mortality rates did not significantly differ between ST-elevation MI and non-ST-elevation MI.[329] The substantial increase in late mortality and reinfarction associated with non-ST-elevation MI underscores the need for close follow-up and secondary prevention measures.

Pitfall: Underuse of GP IIb/IIIa inhibitors in high-risk patients with non-ST-elevation ACS

Randomized clinical trials have consistently demonstrated significant reductions in death or MI with a favorable safety profile when intravenous GP IIb/IIIa inhibitors are added to conventional therapy for patients with non-ST-elevation ACS and positive cardiac troponins (Table 9.2, p. 82). A recent registry study demonstrated that hospitals adhering to use of GP IIb/IIIa inhibitors in high-risk patients had lower mortality rates in non-ST-elevation ACS.

Pitfall: Underuse of ACE inhibitors in acute MI

Randomized trials support early administration of ACE inhibitors to all patients with acute MI regardless of LV function or heart failure symptoms. Oral ACE inhibitors should be initiated once reperfusion has occurred and blood pressure has stabilized, usually no sooner than 6 hours after presentation, and then titrated upward over 12-24 hours. ACE inhibitors should be continued long term in patients with heart failure, left ventricular dysfunction (EF < 0.40), hypertension, or diabetes, and possibly for all patients based on a 22% reduction in stroke, MI, or death at 5 years in the HOPE trial.[63]

Pitfall: Underuse of beta-blockers following acute MI

Beta-blocker therapy is associated with a significant reduction in mortality following acute MI.[330-332] The benefit is seen across many subgroups, including patients with conditions previously considered contraindications to beta-blockers (e.g., heart failure, pulmonary disease, diabetes, advanced age). Diabetics demonstrate twice the mortality benefit of beta-blocker therapy post-MI compared with nondiabetics. Despite marked benefits, only one-third of patients with acute MI receive beta-blockers.[333] Unless there is an absolute contraindication, all patients should be treated with a beta-blocker early after MI. Patients with relative contraindications (e.g., mild obstructive airway disease) can be started on a low dose of a short-acting beta-blocker, with cautious upward titration.

Pitfall: Routine use of IV nitroglycerin in acute MI to the exclusion of other more effective drugs

Existing data support the use of IV nitroglycerin for 24-48 hours in patients with anterior MI, heart failure, persistent ischemia, or hypertension. The usefulness of this medication has not been demonstrated for patients without these clinical features.[334-336] A drawback to the routine use of IV nitroglycerin is that it may preclude the use of more effective therapies, such as beta-blockers and ACE inhibitors, due to its blood pressure lowering effects. IV nitroglycerin is contraindicated in preload-dependent conditions (e.g., right ventricular infarction) and within 24 hours of sildenafil (Viagra), due to the risk of profound hypotension. There is no evidence to support the use of IV nitroglycerin beyond 48 hours in the absence of recurrent ischemia or persistent pulmonary edema.

Pitfall: Failure to treat ACS patients indefinitely with aspirin

Despite a 40% reduction in the risk of in-hospital death, many patients with ACS either do not receive or experience substantial delays in receiving aspirin. In ISIS-2, the mortality benefit of aspirin for acute MI was comparable to fibrinolytic therapy.[337] In addition, long term therapy with aspirin reduces vascular mortality by 17%, stroke by 30%, and recurrent infarction by 30% in patients with prior MI. Despite these convincing data, in one study nearly half of the patients presenting to an emergency room with acute MI did not receive aspirin therapy.[338] All MI patients without a serious aspirin allergy should receive aspirin 81-325 mg (PO) q24h indefinitely.

Pitfall: Failure to discuss smoking cessation regularly and systematically with patients

Continued cigarette smoking is a major risk factor for recurrent events in patients with coronary artery disease, and less than one-third of smokers quit smoking following an acute coronary event. Regular and systematic discussion of the importance of smoking cessation can increase the discontinuation rate to almost 60% and is a critical component of the care of smokers. Even a single physician recommendation to quit smoking has a significant impact on the likelihood of successful abstinence. Patients who experience difficulty quitting should be offered counseling and nicotine preparations or bupropion hydrochloride (Zyban).

Pitfall: Failure to recognize and treat depression following MI

Major depression occurs in up to 25% of patients after MI and has been associated with an increased risk for malignant ventricular arrhythmias and death, possibly due to altered autonomic tone.[325] Major depression should be distinguished from minor depressive symptoms, which are common after MI and are typically short-lived. Major depression is defined by a depressed mood or loss of interest in nearly all activities for a minimum of 2 weeks, plus at least 3 of the following symptoms: insomnia or hypersomnia; feelings of worthlessness or excessive guilt; fatigue or loss of energy; impaired ability to think or concentrate; significant change in appetite; psychomotor agitation or retardation; recurrent thoughts of death or suicide.[325] For patients with moderate or severe symptoms who are unlikely to recover in 2-4 weeks with support and encouragement, a trial of selective serotonin reuptake inhibitors may improve psychosocial functioning, although their impact on survival is unknown. Tricyclic antidepressants should generally be avoided due to the increased risk of postural hypotension, arrhythmias, and conduction abnormalities.[325] To help identify depression in a likely patient, the following two questions should be asked: Do you have little interest or pleasure in doing things you usually enjoy? Are you feeling down, depressed, or helpless?

Pitfall: Failure to risk stratify ACS patients when determining the need for cardiac catheterization during hospitalization
Substantial worldwide variation in cardiac catheterization rates exists despite little improvement in clinical outcomes associated with higher rates of angiography. Early angiography efforts should be focused on patients with recurrent ischemia, advanced age, left ventricular dysfunction, heart failure, or a high likelihood of multivessel disease.

Section 7

DRUG SUMMARIES

This section contains prescribing information for drugs used in the management of acute coronary syndromes, as compiled from a variety of sources. The recommendations are offered as a general guidelines, not specific instructions for individual patients. Clinical judgment should always guide the physician in the selection, dosing, and duration of drug therapy for individual patients. Unless otherwise stated, the dosing recommendations apply to patients with normal renal and hepatic function, not to patients with renal dysfunction, hepatic insufficiency, or other circumstances that may require dosing adjustment. Not all medications have been accepted by the U.S. Food and Drug Administration for indications cited in this section, and drug recommendations are not necessarily limited to indications in the package insert. The use of any drug should be preceded by careful review of the package insert, which provides indications and dosing approved by the U.S. Food and Drug Administration. The information provided is not exhaustive, and the reader is referred to other drug information references and the manufacturer's product literature for further information. Clinical use of the information provided and any consequences that may arise from its use are the responsibilities of the prescribing physician. The authors, editors, and publisher do not warrant or guarantee the information contained in this section, and do not assume and expressly disclaim any liability for errors or omissions or any consequences that may occur from such.

Chapter 16

Drug Summaries

Drug therapy reduces the risk of reinfarction, stroke, and cardiovascular death by limiting infarct size, preventing and treating thrombotic, mechanical, and electrical complications, and halting the progression of atherosclerosis (Table 16.1). This section details acute and chronic medical therapy for ACS.

Table 16.1. Medical Therapy for ACS

	Beneficial Effect	Possible Detrimental Effect
Acute therapy *All patients*	• Aspirin • Heparin • Beta-blockers • ACE inhibitors • Clopidogrel for stenting • IV nitrates for large MI*	• Immediate-release nifedipine • Prophylactic lidocaine • Nitrates for RV infarction or within 24 hours of sildenafil (Viagra)
ST-elevation ACS	• Fibrinolytic therapy • GP IIb/IIIa inhibitors as adjuncts to PCI*	• See "all patients"
Non-ST-elevation ACS	• Clopidogrel • GP IIb/IIIa inhibitors • Enoxaparin	• Fibrinolytic therapy • See "all patients"
Chronic therapy (> 48-72 hours)	• Aspirin • Clopidogrel for non-ST-elevation ACS and for stenting • Beta-blockers • ACE inhibitors • Statins • Warfarin for mobile LV thrombus* or AF • Diltiazem or verapamil for non-Q-wave MI without pulmonary congestion*	• Hormone replacement therapy during 1st year

* Possible benefit, AF = atrial fibrillation, RV = right ventricular

ACE Inhibitors

Indications and Dose: <u>Acute MI within the first 24 hours; hypertension; heart failure; LV dysfunction:</u> Start PO at low-dose as soon as patient is stabilized from MI (after lytics/PCI and blood pressure has stabilized, no sooner than 6 hours post-MI); titrate upward over 1-4 days, as tolerated. Doses (PO): *Captopril* 6.25 mg q8h, titrated to 50 mg q8h; *lisinopril* 2.5 mg q24h, titrated to 10-20 mg q24h; *ramipril* 2.5 mg q12h, titrated to 5 mg q12h; *enalapril* 2.5 mg q12h, titrated to 10-20 mg q12h. For patients unable to take PO medications, IV enalapril can be given at 1.25 mg over 5 minutes, then 1.25-5 mg q6h (avoid in first 24 hours). Other ACE inhibitors are probably as effective. For uncomplicated MI with normal LV function, discontinue after 4-6 weeks or consider long-term therapy for secondary prevention. Continue indefinitely if ejection fraction is reduced.

Contraindications: Do not administer if systolic BP < 90-100 mmHg or there are contraindications to ACE inhibitors (e.g., renal failure, bilateral renal artery stenosis, known allergy).

Clinical Trials: Following acute MI, ACE inhibitors reduce the risk of recurrent MI, progression to heart failure, need for rehospitalization, and death (4.6 fewer deaths for every 1000 patients treated).[339] Survival benefit is evident on first day[335,336] and is greatest for patients with anterior MI, prior MI, heart failure, or LV dysfunction (EF < 0.40). In a meta-analysis of ACE inhibitors for LV dysfunction after acute MI, there were 23 fewer deaths for every 1000 patients treated.[340] In HOPE, ramipril (10 mg/d) reduced the risk of MI, stroke, or death by 22% at 5 years in patients with atherosclerotic vascular disease, including those with prior MI.[63]

Comments: Ensure adequate hydration before starting ACE inhibitors. Avoid IV enalaprilat acutely (first 24 hours) due to lack of benefit and possible harm in CONSESUS II.[341]

Adenosine

Indications and Dose:[248] <u>Termination of sinus node reentrant tachycardia, AV nodal reentrant tachycardia, or reentrant tachycardias utilizing an accessory pathway:</u> 6-mg IV bolus over 1-2 seconds. If needed, a 12-mg IV bolus can be given 1-2 minutes later, followed by another 12-mg IV bolus 1-2 minutes after the second dose. Each IV dose should be followed with a rapid saline flush (20 cc) and elevation of the extremity.

Contraindications: Avoid in drug-induced tachycardias, wide QRS tachycardias of unknown origin, and patients taking dipyridamole.

Comments: Does not convert atrial fibrillation, atrial flutter, or VT. Transient side effects include flushing, chest pain, dyspnea, brief asystole, bradycardia, VPCs. Transient sinus bradycardia and VPCs are common after conversion to sinus rhythm.

Dosages assume normal renal and hepatic function, unless otherwise specified. Check other drug references for complete prescribing information, including dosage adjustments, drug interactions, adverse effects, and safety in pregnancy.

Amiodarone

Indications and Dose:[248] <u>Cardiac arrest (VF or pulseless VT):</u> Initial IV bolus of 300 mg. Can repeat 150-mg bolus doses as needed up to a total maximum dose of 2.1 gm in 24 hours. <u>Recurrent/refractory VF/VT, life-threatening VF, hemodynamically unstable VT, stable wide-complex tachycardia:</u> Begin with IV infusion of 150 mg over no less than 10 minutes. This may be followed by an infusion of 1 mg/min x 6 hours, then a maintenance infusion of 0.5 mg/min thereafter until the switch to oral amiodarone can be made. Additional bolus infusions of 150 mg over no less than 10 minutes can be administered for breakthrough events. <u>Oral dosing for life-threatening recurrent VF or recurrent hemodynamically-unstable VT not responsive to other antiarrhythmics:</u> Loading dose of 800-1600 mg/d x 1-3 weeks (occasionally longer) until the arrhythmia is controlled or prominent side effects occur. The dose should then be reduced to 600-800 mg/d x 1 month, followed by the usual maintenance dose of 400 mg/d. Amiodarone should be administered once daily (or in divided doses with meals for total daily doses ≥ 800 mg or GI intolerance). Use lowest effective dose.

Contraindications: Severe sinus node dysfunction causing marked sinus bradycardia; second- or third-degree AV block; symptomatic bradyarrhythmias without a functioning pacemaker. Use with caution in renal failure and with other drugs that prolong the QT interval.

Clinical Trials: Amiodarone reduced VF or arrhythmic death in patients with acute MI and frequent PVCs[342] or LV dysfunction (EF < 0.40),[343] but had no effect on total mortality.

Comments: Not recommended chronically unless the risk of recurrent hemodynamically-unstable ventricular arrhythmias is high. The most common serious side effects include hypotension, bradycardia, AV block, torsade de pointes (< 2%), ARDS (2%), and negative inotropic effects in some. Exclude amiodarone-induced hyperthyroidism with new signs of arrhythmia. Therapy should be initiated in the hospital, and gradual withdrawal of other antiarrhythmic drugs should be attempted when starting amiodarone. For monitoring during chronic therapy, baseline work-up should include a chest x-ray, pulmonary function tests (including diffusion capacity), and thyroid function tests; physical examination, thyroid function tests, liver function tests, and chest x-ray should be repeated every 3-6 months during therapy. Plasma concentrations (normal: 1-2.5 mcg/mL) may be helpful in evaluating non-responsiveness or unexpected severe toxicity. Patients should be monitored closely after dosage adjustments due to amiodarone's long half-life (9-44 days). Amiodarone can increase serum levels of digoxin, quinidine, procainamide, flecainide, cyclosporine, and warfarin (follow prothrombin times closely). Phenytoin

---

Dosages assume normal renal and hepatic function, unless otherwise specified. Check other drug references for complete prescribing information, including dosage adjustments, drug interactions, adverse effects, and safety in pregnancy.

and cholestyramine can reduce amiodarone levels. Amiodarone can also be used as an adjunct to cardioversion for SVT, for rate control of ectopic or multifocal atrial tachycardia in patients with preserved LV function, and for rate control of atrial fibrillation or flutter when other therapies are ineffective. Amiodarone should only be used by physicians with access to all modalities used for treating and monitoring recurrent life-threatening ventricular arrhythmias.

Aspirin

Indications and Dose: <u>All ACS patients:</u> 162-325 mg of a nonenteric-coated preparation chewed acutely, followed by 75-325 mg (PO) q24h of an enteric- or nonenteric-coated preparation long term. Rectal suppositories (325 mg) can be used for patients unable to take oral medications.

Contraindications: Active bleeding; aspirin allergy; severe hypertension; active peptic ulcer disease. Not recommended in the third trimester of pregnancy. Can precipitate gout.

Clinical Trials: Aspirin reduces vascular death, MI, and stroke by 29% at 1 month and 24% at 2 years following acute MI and by 36% at 6 months following unstable angina.[60,344] Aspirin enhances coronary reperfusion after fibrinolytic therapy, and it reduces the risk of reocclusion after fibrinolytic therapy,[345] PCI,[153] and CABG. It has been estimated that aspirin prevents 24 deaths, 12 reinfarctions, and 2 strokes for every 1000 patients treated post-MI.[346]

Comments: Aspirin exerts its antiplatelet effects by blocking the formation of thromboxane A_2 through irreversible acetylation of platelet cyclooxygenase. Enzyme inhibition lasts for the lifespan of the platelet (~ 10 days). Aspirin does not prevent platelet adhesion or platelet aggregation in response to ADP, collagen, thrombin, or epinephrine. Aspirin blocks the formation of bradykinin, raising concern over a possible aspirin-ACE inhibitor antagonism. However, most studies indicate that this interaction is not clinically relevant,[347,348] and that aspirin should not be withheld in patients receiving ACE inhibitors. Long-term administration of ibuprofen (but not acetaminophen, rofecoxib, or diclofenac) may interfere with the cardiovascular protective effects of aspirin.[349] Buccal absorption of chewed aspirin is the fastest route for platelet inhibition. Enteric-coated preparations should be avoided acutely due to delays in GI absorption and platelet inhibition. Up to 10% of patients with coronary artery disease are aspirin-resistant.[157]

Atropine

Indications and Dose: <u>Ventricular asystole; pulseless electrical activity:</u> 1 mg IV push (may repeat). <u>Symptomatic sinus bradycardia or intranodal (Mobitz type I) AV block; nausea and vomiting caused by morphine:</u> 0.5-1.0 mg. This may be repeated up to a total dose of 3

Dosages assume normal renal and hepatic function, unless otherwise specified. Check other drug references for complete prescribing information, including dosage adjustments, drug interactions, adverse effects, and safety in pregnancy.

mg. Tracheal dose/route: 1-2.5 mg in 10-25 cc normal saline.

Contraindications: Use with caution in ACS (increased heart rate can provoke myocardial ischemia, acute MI, and rarely VT or VF).

Comments: Atropine can worsen infranodal (Mobitz type II) second-degree AV block. Low doses (< 0.5 mg) can cause paradoxical slowing of heart rate.

Beta-Blockers, Acute

Indications and Dose: All ACS patients: Start IV in high-risk patients (e.g., acute MI, ongoing pain, dynamic ECG changes), then switch to PO therapy. For intermediate- or low-risk patients with unstable angina and no pain, it is acceptable to start with PO therapy. *Metoprolol*: 5 mg (IV) over 1-2 minutes, repeated every 5 minutes for a total initial dose of 15 mg. Follow in 15 minutes with 50 mg (PO) q12h x 24h, then 100 mg (PO) q12h, as tolerated. Initial doses can be reduced to 1-2 mg if a conservative regimen is desired. *Atenolol*: 5 mg (IV) over 5 minutes, repeated 5 minutes later x 1. Follow in 10 minutes, if tolerated, with 50 mg (PO) q12h. *Esmolol*: 0.1 mg/kg/min (IV) infusion, titrated in increments of 0.05 mg/kg/min every 5-15 minutes (as tolerated by blood pressure) until the desired therapeutic response is achieved, limiting symptoms develop, or a dose of 0.25 mg/kg/min is reached. For more rapid onset of action, a loading dose of 0.5 mg/kg can be given IV over 2-5 minutes followed by the usual maintenance dose. Other beta-blockers without intrinsic sympathomimetic activity (ISA) are probably equally as effective.

Contraindications (relative): Systolic BP < 100 mmHg; HR < 50 bpm; severe, decompensated heart failure; PR interval > 0.24 seconds; greater than first-degree AV block or sick sinus syndrome without a functioning pacemaker; history of clinically-important bronchospasm. Use with caution in diabetics with hypoglycemia. Concurrent use with verapamil or diltiazem can result in severe hypotension or heart failure.

Clinical Trials: For acute MI, early administration of beta-blockers limits infarct size,[350] reduces ventricular fibrillation and cardiac rupture,[351] decreases reinfarction and intracranial hemorrhage after fibrinolytic therapy,[352] and reduces mortality by 15% within the first week.[353] Mortality benefit is evident by the end of day 1 and is sustained thereafter, emphasizing the importance of early administration. For unstable angina, beta-blockers reduce MI by 13%.[354] Beta-blockers control ischemic pain in some patients.

Comments: Monitor heart rate, blood pressure, ECG; evaluate lungs for rales and wheezing. Beta-blockers should be used very cautiously, if at all, in patients with severe COPD. For mild wheezing or COPD, consider using a low-dose of a beta-1-selective agent (e.g., metoprolol 2.5 mg IV or 12.5 mg PO).

Dosages assume normal renal and hepatic function, unless otherwise specified. Check other drug references for complete prescribing information, including dosage adjustments, drug interactions, adverse effects, and safety in pregnancy.

Beta-Blockers, Chronic

Indications and Dose: All ACS patients, except those with symptomatic bradycardia, high-grade heart block, decompensated heart failure, or significant bronchospasm: Timolol 10 mg (PO) q12h, atenolol 50-200 mg (PO) q24h, metoprolol 50-200 mg (PO) q12h, or another beta-blocker. Treat to target heart rate of 50-60 bpm. Continue for at least 2 years, even after successful PCI or CABG.

Clinical Trials: Long-term therapy reduces the risk of reinfarction and death (primarily sudden death) by 25-45% at 1 year[330,331] and by 20% up to 6 years after MI,[332] especially in high-risk patients with anterior MI. Benefits are also apparent in patients with conditions often considered as contraindications to beta-blocker therapy: advanced age, pulmonary disease, heart failure.[333]

Comments: There is no difference between nonselective and selective agents, although beta-blockers without intrinsic sympathomimetic activity (ISA) may be more effective than beta-blockers with ISA.[335] Beta-blockers should be gradually withdrawn over 1-2 weeks, not stopped abruptly.

Calcium Antagonists

Indications and Dose: Relief of ongoing or recurrent ischemia when beta-blockers are contraindicated or ineffective; ACS due to variant angina or cocaine use; possibly for non-Q-wave MI with preserved LV function: Diltiazem 120-320 mg/d or verapamil 120-480 mg/d PO in single or divided doses depending on the preparation. If used for non-Q-wave-MI, calcium antagonists should be started early (2-5 days) and continued for up to 1 year. Calcium antagonists that do not slow heart rate (e.g., nifedipine, nicardipine) must be used in conjunction with a beta-blocker. For ACS due to suspected cocaine use, consider diltiazem 20 mg IV. To slow the ventricular response to atrial fibrillation/flutter: *Diltiazem:* Initial IV bolus of 0.25 mg/kg (~ 20 mg) over 2 minutes. If response is inadequate, a second bolus of 0.35 mg/kg (~ 25 mg) can be given 15 minutes later. For continued reduction of ventricular rate (up to 24 hours), an IV infusion of 5-15 mg/hr can be started immediately after the bolus and titrated to heart rate. Infusion rates > 15 mg/hr are not recommended. *Verapamil:* see dose for paroxysmal SVT, below. To terminate paroxysmal SVT after adenosine in patients with good blood pressure and preserved LV function: *Diltiazem:* Initial IV bolus of 0.25 mg/kg IV over 2 minutes. If SVT persists, a second bolus of 0.35 mg/kg can be given 15 minutes later. *Verapamil:* Initial IV bolus of 2.5-5.0 mg over 1-2 minutes (3 minutes in the elderly); peak effect in 3-5 minutes. If needed, a second bolus of 5-10 mg can be given 15-30 minutes after the first dose or 5-mg bolus doses can be repeated every 15 minutes up to a total cumulative dose of 30 mg.

Contraindications: Diltiazem and verapamil should be used with extreme

---

Dosages assume normal renal and hepatic function, unless otherwise specified. Check other drug references for complete prescribing information, including dosage adjustments, drug interactions, adverse effects, and safety in pregnancy.

caution, if at all, with IV beta-blockers or in patients with heart failure, severe LV dysfunction, or sick sinus syndrome or greater than first-degree AV block without a functioning pacemaker. Neither agent should be used IV to slow the ventricular response to atrial fibrillation or flutter in Wolff-Parkinson-White syndrome (increased risk of VF) or to treat VT (increased risk of fatal hypotension). Rapid-release, short-acting nifedipine and other calcium antagonists that do not slow heart rate must be used with a beta-blocker due to the increased risk of reinfarction and death.[356-358]

Clinical Trials (Acute MI): Diltiazem reduced early reinfarction and recurrent angina in non-Q-wave MI [359,360] and in ST-elevation MI treated with fibrinolytic therapy,[361] but increased mortality in patients with heart failure or severe LV dysfunction.[359] One report indicated a possible role for verapamil plus ACE inhibitors for LV dysfunction post-MI.[362]

Comments: The primary benefit of calcium antagonists in unstable angina is the prevention and relief of ischemia. Side effects include hypotension, heart failure, and bradycardia. Verapamil can increase serum digitalis levels. IV calcium chloride (8-16 mg/kg for overdose; 2-4 mg/kg for prophylaxis) can be used to restore/prevent the drop in blood pressure associated with calcium antagonists. Amlodipine or felodipine can be safely administered to patients with chronic LV dysfunction, but their role in acute MI awaits definition. Verapamil can also be used to slow the ventricular rate in multifocal atrial tachycardia.

Clopidogrel

Indications and Dose: Non-ST-elevation ACS: 300 mg (PO) loading dose, in conjunction with aspirin, started as soon as possible on admission and continued at 75 mg (PO) q24h for at least 1 month and possibly for 9 months (see "precautions"). Coronary stenting: 300 mg (PO) loading dose prior to PCI followed by 75 mg (PO) q24h x 1 year.[398] Aspirin-allergic or intolerant patients: 75 mg (PO) q24h long term.

Precautions: Use with caution in conjunction with NSAIDs or warfarin (increased risk of bleeding). Clopidogrel should be discontinued 5-7 days prior to CABG, if possible, to minimize the risk of perioperative bleeding. In patients submitted for urgent angiography and revascularization, it is reasonable to withhold clopidogrel until it is known that CABG will not be required.

Clinical Trials: In CURE[162] and PCI-CURE,[163] dual antiplatelet therapy with aspirin plus clopidogrel resulted in 20-30% reductions in cardiovascular death, MI, or stroke in non-ST-elevation ACS compared to aspirin alone (p. 77). In CAPRIE,[166] clopidogrel showed a small (8.7%) but significant relative reduction in ischemic stroke, MI, or vascular death at 1.9 years compared to aspirin in high-risk patients with recent ischemic stroke, recent MI, or symptomatic peripheral arterial disease (p. 78).

....

Dosages assume normal renal and hepatic function, unless otherwise specified. Check other drug references for complete prescribing information, including dosage adjustments, drug interactions, adverse effects, and safety in pregnancy.

Comments: Clopidogrel irreversibly modifies the platelet ADP receptor and interferes with ADP-dependent activation of the platelet GP IIb/IIIa receptor but does not inhibit the arachidonic acid pathway. The safety profile of clopidogrel is similar to low-dose aspirin, with a rare incidence of thrombotic thrombocytopenia purpura (TTP) (11 cases in 3 million patients in one report).[167] The most frequent side effects include diarrhea, rash, and pruritus. The risk of granulocytopenia is not increased.

Dobutamine

Indications and Dose:[248] Acute heart failure without shock; hemodynamically-significant RV infarction not responding to volume loading: 2-30 mcg/kg/min IV infusion. Doses up to 40 mcg/kg/min have been used. Use lowest effective dose, as tachycardia is more likely to develop at higher doses. Titrate infusion so heart rate does not increase > 10%. Taper gradually upon discontinuation.
Contraindications: Avoid in cardiogenic shock, severe aortic stenosis, idiopathic hypertrophic subaortic stenosis (IHSS), sulfite allergy (possible anaphylaxis).
Comments: Dobutamine is a potent inotropic agent with mild peripheral vasodilating effects; the net hemodynamic effect is similar to dopamine plus a vasodilator. Tolerance can occur with prolonged (> 24 hour) use, requiring an increase in dose. Myocardial ischemia and arrhythmias can occur if tachycardia is induced. Dobutamine is inactivated if mixed with solutions containing sodium bicarbonate. Hemodynamic monitoring with a pulmonary artery catheter is recommended during dobutamine infusions.

Dopamine

Indications and Dose:[248] Severe hypotension: Initial IV infusion of 1-5 mcg/kg/min, titrated based on blood pressure. Usually effective below rates of 20 mcg/kg/min. Use lowest effective dose, as tachycardia and systemic/splanchnic vasoconstriction are more likely to develop at higher doses. Taper gradually upon discontinuation; additional IV fluids may be required during taper.
Contraindications: Avoid in patients with pheochromocytoma, VF, sulfite allergy (possible anaphylaxis).
Comments: Dopamine can constrict pulmonary veins, which can increase pulmonary capillary wedge pressure and worsen pulmonary congestion despite improving cardiac output; this effect can be offset with concomitant use of a vasodilator (e.g., nitroglycerin, nitroprusside). Tachyphylaxis can occur with prolonged use, requiring an increase in dose. Only 10% of the usual dopamine dose should be given to patients receiving MAO inhibitors (MAO inhibitors can increase the pressor response to dopamine by 6-20-fold). Subcutaneous extravasation can cause skin sloughing

----

Dosages assume normal renal and hepatic function, unless otherwise specified. Check other drug references for complete prescribing information, including dosage adjustments, drug interactions, adverse effects, and safety in pregnancy.

and should be treated with local infiltration of phentolamine. Dopamine can also be used for symptomatic bradycardia unresponsive to atropine. Dopamine is inactivated when mixed with solutions containing sodium bicarbonate. Hemodynamic monitoring with a pulmonary artery catheter is recommended during dopamine infusions.

Epinephrine

Indications:[248] Asystole; pulseless electrical activity; VF or pulseless VT resistant to defibrillation; severe hypotension; symptomatic bradycardia after atropine.

Dose: Cardiac arrest: 1 mg (10 cc of 1:10,000 solution) IV bolus or 2 mg (diluted in 10 cc normal saline) via endotracheal tube. May be repeated every 3-5 minutes. Higher doses (up to 0.2 mg/kg) are not routinely recommended but can be considered if the initial doses are ineffective. Each IV bolus should be followed by a saline flush (20 cc). Profound bradycardia or hypotension: 2-10 mcg/min IV infusion.

Comments: Epinephrine can precipitate myocardial ischemia even at low doses. Epinephrine may be inactivated if mixed in the same solution as bicarbonate. If subcutaneous extravasation occurs, tissue necrosis can develop. Intracardiac injections should only be used during open cardiac massage or when other routes are unavailable. Inadvertent overdose can be counteracted by phentolamine. Discontinue if paradoxical worsening of respiratory function occurs in sulfite-allergic patients (epinephrine contains sulfite).

Fibrinolytic Therapy (tPA, rPA, TNK-tPA, streptokinase)

Indications and Dose: Acute MI < 12 hours with ST-elevation or LBBB (new or presumably new) on ECG and no contraindications to fibrinolytic therapy: See pp. 45-46 for dosing regimens.

Clinical Trials: Randomized trials demonstrated a 21% relative risk reduction in 35-day mortality compared to standard medical therapy (Chapter 5). Mortality benefits are greatest when lytics are given within 6 hours, intermediate at 7-12 hours, and there is little or no benefit after 12 hours unless there is persistent ischemia or recurrent ST-elevation. All patient subgroups benefit, regardless of gender, race, or age, but patients with hypotension, tachycardia, diabetes mellitus, or prior MI derive the greatest benefit.

Comments: Conversion of single-chain plasminogen to double-chain plasmin by fibrinolytic agents results in degradation of fibrin and dissolution of clot. See pp. 40-55 for fibrinolytic agents, dosing regimens, adjunctive pharmacotherapy, contraindications, and management of complications.

Dosages assume normal renal and hepatic function, unless otherwise specified. Check other drug references for complete prescribing information, including dosage adjustments, drug interactions, adverse effects, and safety in pregnancy.

Furosemide

Indications and Dose: <u>Acute treatment of pulmonary congestion associated with LV dysfunction:</u> 20-40 mg IV over 1-2 minutes. If no response, doses up to 2 mg/kg may be needed.

Comments: Diuretic effect peaks at 30 minutes and lasts for 6 hours. Reductions in venous return and central venous pressure occur before the onset of diuresis. Furosemide can induce hypotension, especially in patients with hypovolemia, RV infarction, or concurrent use of morphine or vasodilators. Potassium, calcium, and magnesium levels should be monitored to minimize the risk of arrhythmias. Furosemide can induce allergic reactions in sulfa-allergic patients.

Glucose-Insulin-Potassium (GIK)

Indications: Acute ST-elevation MI.

Dose: Many different regimens.

Clinical Trials: Shown to reduce mortality in diabetics with acute MI at 1 year in DIGAMI.[363] Meta-analysis of 15 trials demonstrated a 28% reduction in hospital mortality.[364] Recent GIPS study of 940 patients failed to show a reduction in mortality, but subset without heart failure (Killip Class I) appeared to benefit.[364a]

Comments: May decrease reperfusion injury by blocking the formation of free fatty acids and free radicals.

GP IIb/IIIa Inhibitors (abciximab, eptifibatide, tirofiban)

Indications: Eptifibatide or tirofiban as primary medical therapy for non-ST-elevation ACS in patients at high risk of thrombotic complications (e.g., ongoing ischemic pain, elevated cardiac troponins, dynamic ST-segment changes). Abciximab, eptifibatide, or tirofiban as an adjunct to PCI for non-ST-elevation ACS.

Dose: See Table 9.3, p. 83.

Clinical Trials: In a meta-analysis of 14 large-scale, randomized, placebo-controlled trials, GP IIb/IIIa inhibitors resulted in a significant reduction in death or MI at 30 days when used as an adjunct to PCI (36%; $p < 0.001$) or as primary medical therapy for non-ST-elevation ACS (9%; $p = 0.015$) (Table 9.2, p. 82). Risk reduction was greatest for troponin-positive patients. The role for GP IIb/IIIa inhibitors in conjunction with low-dose fibrinolytic therapy for ST-elevation MI has recently been evaluated in ASSENT-3 and GUSTO-V (pp. 55-56).

Comments: See pp. 79-84 for dosing and administration guidelines, use of adjunctive aspirin and heparin, management of complications, and trial results.

Dosages assume normal renal and hepatic function, unless otherwise specified. Check other drug references for complete prescribing information, including dosage adjustments, drug interactions, adverse effects, and safety in pregnancy.

Heparin, Low-Molecular-Weight (LMWH)

Indications and Dose: <u>Primary medical therapy for non-ST-elevation ACS:</u> Enoxaparin 1 mg/kg SQ q12h. The optimal duration of therapy is unknown, but most patients receive enoxaparin for 2-8 days. Decrease dose by 25-50% for significant renal impairment. <u>Adjunct to PCI:</u> Enoxaparin 0.75 mg/kg IV if a GP IIb/IIIa inhibitor is to be used; 1 mg/kg IV if *no* GP IIb/IIIa inhibitor is planned. If patient has been treated with SQ enoxaparin and the last SQ dose is < 8 hours, no additional enoxaparin is required prior to PCI; if the last SQ dose is > 8 hours, an additional 0.3 mg/kg IV should be given just before PCI.

Clinical Trials: As primary medical therapy for non-ST-elevation ACS, two enoxaparin vs. UFH trials (ESSENCE, TIMI 11b)[186,187] showed a significant 20% reduction in death or MI at 1 and 6 weeks with enoxaparin (Table 9.5, p. 87). In contrast, dalteparin (FRIC)[189] and nadroparin (FRAXIS)[190] failed to show benefit over UFH. As an adjunct to PCI, observational studies (NICE-1, NICE-3, NICE-4)[192-194] and randomized trials (ACUTE II, CRUISE, INTERACT)[195-197] have shown enoxaparin to be a safe and effective alternative to UFH for procedural anticoagulation (with or without GP IIb/IIIa inhibitors); compared to UFH, enoxaparin was more convenient to use and resulted in similar rates of ischemic events and major bleeding complications. In the ASSENT 3 trial of enoxaparin vs. UFH as an adjunct to TNK-tPA for ST-elevation MI, enoxaparin resulted in better event-free survival at 30 days (Table 5.6, p. 55).[122]

Comments: LMWHs are homogeneous glycosaminoglycans with a mean molecular weight of 4000-6000 formed by controlled enzymatic or chemical depolymerization of unfractionated heparin (UFH).[181] Advantages over UFH include better inhibition of thrombin generation (higher anti-Xa to anti-IIa activity), lack of need to monitor aPTT (excellent bioavailability results in reliable anticoagulation), ease of administration (subcutaneous route), lack of inhibition by platelet factor IV, and less heparin-induced thrombocytopenia. In clinical trials, LMWHs were associated with more minor bleeding than UFH but no increase in major bleeding complications. See pp. 85-91 for use of enoxaparin in non-ST-elevation ACS, monitoring, and management of complications. To minimize the risk of vascular bleeding, vascular access sheaths should remain in place for 6-8 hours after the last enoxaparin dose, and the next enoxaparin dose should be given no sooner than 6-8 hours after sheath removal.[198] Hemoglobin, hematocrit, and platelet counts should be monitored daily, and enoxaparin should be discontinued if the platelet count falls below 100,000 mm³.

Dosages assume normal renal and hepatic function, unless otherwise specified. Check other drug references for complete prescribing information, including dosage adjustments, drug interactions, adverse effects, and safety in pregnancy.

Heparin, Unfractionated (UFH)

Indications and Dose:

Adjunct to tPA, rPA, TNK-tPA: 60-70 U/kg IV bolus (max. 5000 U) followed by 12-15 U/kg/hr IV maintenance infusion (max. 1000 U/hr), adjusted to aPTT of 1.5-2.5 times control (50-75 sec) x 48 hours (or until angiography or longer in patients at high risk of thromboembolism). Adjunct to streptokinase for patients at high risk of thromboembolism (large anterior MI, low cardiac output, atrial fibrillation, previous embolus, LV thrombus): IV infusion (as for tPA) without a bolus, starting 4-6 hours after streptokinase or when the aPTT < 2-3 times control. UFH is not routinely required with streptokinase in low-risk patients, as streptokinase has anticoagulant properties, including generation of fibrin degradation products and depletion of clotting factors V and VIII. Primary medical therapy for non-ST-elevation ACS: IV bolus plus infusion as for tPA, above. For patients receiving GP IIb/IIIa inhibitors, the dose of UFH used with eptifibatide in PURSUIT was 5000 U IV bolus plus 1000 U/hr titrated to aPTT of 50-70 sec; for weight ≤ 70 kg, the dose was reduced to 60 U/kg IV bolus plus 12 U/kg/hr IV infusion. In PRISM-PLUS, the dose of UFH used with tirofiban was 5000 U IV bolus plus 1000 U/hr IV infusion titrated to aPTT ~ 2 times control. During PCI: 60-100 U/kg IV bolus to achieve an intraprocedural ACT of 300-350 seconds. When a GP IIb/IIIa inhibitor is used, a 60 U/kg IV bolus is given to achieve an intraprocedural ACT of 200-250 seconds. All patients not being treated with IV heparin during periods of prolonged immobilization: 7500 units (SQ) q12h (or enoxaparin 1 mg/kg SQ q12h)

Contraindications: Active bleeding; severe, uncontrolled hypertension; recent intracranial, intraspinal, or eye surgery; heparin-induced thrombocytopenia (HIT). Caution in patients with bacterial endocarditis or potential sources of severe bleeding.

Clinical Trials: Compared to aspirin alone, IV heparin reduces the risk of death or reinfarction by 30-50% in non-ST-elevation ACS[365-369] and by 17-22% in ST-elevation ACS.[370] IV heparin is probably necessary for the 1% mortality benefit associated with accelerated tPA vs. streptokinase,[371] but routine heparin is probably not necessary with streptokinase due to an increased risk of bleeding without a reduction in death or reinfarction.[113,372,373] Subcutaneous heparin has been shown to reduce the incidence of mural thrombus post-MI by 58-72%.[374,375]

Comments: Heparin is a heterogeneous mucopolysaccharide that binds to antithrombin to potentiate the inhibition of clotting factors IIa (thrombin) and Xa.[181] Heparin binds to plasma proteins, endothelial cells, and macrophages, resulting in variable anticoagulant effects and the need to monitor aPTT or ACT. Other disadvantages include inhibition by platelet factor IV, inability to inactivate

Dosages assume normal renal and hepatic function, unless otherwise specified. Check other drug references for complete prescribing information, including dosage adjustments, drug interactions, adverse effects, and safety in pregnancy.

clot-bound thrombin, and development of heparin-induced thrombocytopenia (HIT).[376] The optimal duration of heparin therapy is unknown, but most ACS patients receive treatment for 2-5 days. (No additional heparin is usually given after successful PCI.) aPTT levels should be obtained 6 hours after starting or changing the heparin dose (see Table 5.4, p. 49, for dose adjustment nomogram); when 2 consecutive aPTT levels are therapeutic, they should be checked once daily thereafter, along with hemoglobin, hematocrit, and platelet counts. The role for abrupt vs. gradual discontinuation of IV heparin infusions is under investigation (possible hyperthrombotic state following abrupt discontinuation). IV anticoagulation in patients with HIT may be achieved with argatroban at 2 mcg/kg/min (p. 91), lepirudin at 0.4 mg/kg (max. 44 mg) bolus over 15-20 seconds followed by 0.15 mg/kg/hr (max. 16.5 mg/hr) (p. 91),[377] or bivalirudin (IV bolus of 0.75 mg/kg prior to balloon inflation followed immediately by an IV infusion of 2.5 mg/kg/hr continued up to 4 hours post-procedure. If ACT < 225 seconds 5 minutes after bolus, additional 0.3 mg/kg boluses are given as needed until ACT = 225 seconds).

Ibutilide

Indications and Dose: Termination of atrial fibrillation or flutter: 1 mg IV over 10 minutes (or 0.01 mg/kg IV if < 60 kg). If the arrhythmia does not terminate within 10 minutes after the initial infusion, a second 10-minute infusion may be given of either 50% of the initial dose or the full initial dose.

Comments: Most patients who convert to sinus rhythm do so within 30 minutes (usual) to 90 minutes. Ventricular arrhythmias (proarrhythmias) occur in 2-5%, especially in patients with LV dysfunction. Continuous ECG monitoring is recommended for 4-6 hours following administration or until the QTc interval returns to baseline.

Lidocaine

Indications and Dose:[248] VF or pulseless VT resistant to defibrillation and epinephrine; hemodynamically-stable VT; hemodynamically-unstable VPCs:
(1) Normal LV function and no hepatic impairment: loading dose of 75 mg IV followed by 50 mg IV every 5 minutes x 3 (total dose 225 mg); maintenance infusion of 2 mg/min. (2) Moderate decrease in LV function: loading dose of 75 mg IV followed by 50 mg IV every 5 minutes x 1 (total dose 125 mg); maintenance infusion of 1 mg/min. (3) Severe decrease in LV function or significant hepatic impairment: loading dose of 50-75 mg IV x 1; maintenance infusion of 0.5 mg/min. A single IV bolus of 1.5 mg/kg is acceptable for cardiac arrest. Tracheal administration: 2-4 mg/kg.

Clinical Trials: Prophylactic lidocaine for acute MI is not recommended (increased risk of death primarily from asystole).[257,378]

Dosages assume normal renal and hepatic function, unless otherwise specified. Check other drug references for complete prescribing information, including dosage adjustments, drug interactions, adverse effects, and safety in pregnancy.

Comments: Monitor for lidocaine toxicity: confusion, drowsiness, respiratory depression, perioral numbness, seizures. May cause bradycardia, sinus arrest. Do not give for ventricular escape beats or rhythm (increased risk of asystole).

Magnesium Sulfate

Indications and Dose: Cardiac arrest due to torsades de pointes: 1-2 gm IV push over 1-2 minutes in 10 cc D_5W. Torsade de pointes (not in cardiac arrest): 1-2 gm in 50-100 cc D_5W IV over 5-60 minutes. Consider an additional 2 gm IV over the next several hours. Regimens vary.

Clinical Trials: Several randomized trials suggested a mortality benefit for IV magnesium for acute MI,[379-383] especially in high-risk patients not receiving reperfusion therapy and in elderly patients following fibrinolysis. In contrast, no benefit was observed in ISIS-4,[335] which enrolled 58,050 patients, although the low mortality rate in control group (7.2%) and late administration of IV magnesium (i.e., after fibrinolytic therapy) were important limitations of this study.[384] Recent results from the NHLBI-sponsored MAGIC trial, which randomized 6213 patients with acute MI to IV magnesium or placebo, failed to show a benefit for magnesium.[384a]

Comments: Magnesium is a coronary vasodilator, has antiplatelet and antiarrhythmic effects, and can prevent calcium overload of reperfused myocytes.[385,386] Magnesium may be of benefit for refractory VT after lidocaine and amiodarone and for life-threatening ventricular arrhythmias due to digitalis toxicity. Not routinely recommended for acute MI unless magnesium deficiency is documented.

Morphine Sulfate

Indications and Dose: Ischemic chest pain; acute pulmonary edema associated with LV dysfunction: 1-5 mg IV over 1-5 minutes, repeated every 5-30 minutes in small increments as needed.

Contraindications: Use with caution in severe, chronic lung disease (increased risk of respiratory depression). Use with caution in RV infarction or volume-depleted patients (may induce hypotension).

Comments: In addition to analgesic properties, morphine dilates peripheral venous and arterial beds, reducing preload, afterload, and myocardial oxygen consumption. Adverse effects include hypoventilation, hypotension, nausea/vomiting. Hypoventilation can be reversed with naloxone (0.4-2.0 mg IV). Hypotension usually responds to leg elevation ± IV saline (200-500 cc bolus in absence of pulmonary congestion). Bradycardia, nausea, vomiting may improve with atropine (0.5-1.0 mg IV).

Nitroglycerin, Acute

Indications and Dose: On initial presentation to control ongoing ischemic pain: Sublingual nitroglycerin tablets (0.4

mg) or aerosol spray every 5 minutes x 3. Aerosol spray should not be shaken (affects metered dose). IV nitroglycerin acutely for persistent ischemic pain despite sublingual nitroglycerin and IV beta-blockers: Initial IV infusion of 10-20 mcg/min. The infusion should be increased by 10 mcg/min every 5 minutes until ischemia is relieved, mean arterial pressure falls by 10% (or 25-30% if hypertensive), heart rate increases by 10 bpm, or pulmonary artery end-diastolic pressure decreases by 10-30%. Do not allow systolic BP to fall below 90 mmHg or heart rate to exceed 110 bpm. Doses in excess of 200 mcg/min are generally not recommended. IV nitroglycerin x 24-48 hours for acute MI or high-risk unstable angina with hypertension, recurrent ischemia, or heart failure: see dose above. **Contraindications:** Systolic BP < 90 mmHg; severe bradycardia (< 50 bpm) or tachycardia; RV infarction; severe hypovolemia; sildenafil (Viagra) use within the previous 24 hours (may cause severe hypotension or MI).

Clinical Trials: IV nitroglycerin reduced infarct size and death in patients treated within 4 hours of anterior MI in a meta-analysis of 10 small trials,[387] but ISIS-4[335] and GISSI-3[336] failed to show a mortality benefit. There are no large randomized trials of IV nitroglycerin for unstable angina.

Comments: Nitroglycerin yields nitric oxide, a smooth muscle relaxant that increases myocardial blood flow and decreases myocardial oxygen consumption. IV administration is preferred over nonparenteral (oral, dermal) routes acutely, due to ease of titration and predictable bioavailability; long-acting oral nitrate preparations should be avoided early. Nitrates should be decreased or discontinued if blood pressure-lowering effects preclude use of beta-blockers/ACE inhibitors. Common side effects include hypotension and headaches. Nitroglycerin can worsen V/Q mismatch and cause hypoxemia in COPD patients who rely on hypoxic pulmonary vasoconstriction to maintain oxygenation. Tolerance (lack of response) to anti-ischemic effects can occur after one day of continuous therapy, requiring an increase in dose or a nitrate-free interval (~ 12 hours). Supplemental antioxidants (e.g., vitamin C) may also prevent nitrate tolerance. Nitrates can reduce the sensitivity to heparin: Higher heparin doses may be needed during nitrate administration and lower heparin doses may be needed once nitrates are stopped (follow ACT/aPTT).

Nitroglycerin, Chronic

Indications and Dose: To prevent recurrent angina: Isosorbide dinitrate sustained-release: start at 40 mg PO qd; may increase to 160 mg qd (18-hour nitrate-free interval is recommended). Isosorbide mononitrate immediate-release (Ismo): 20 mg PO bid (doses given 7 hours apart). Isosorbide mononitrate extended-release (Imdur): 30-60 mg PO q24h titrated to ~ 120 mg q24h.
Clinical Trials: Oral nitrates starting on

Dosages assume normal renal and hepatic function, unless otherwise specified. Check other drug references for complete prescribing information, including dosage adjustments, drug interactions, adverse effects, and safety in pregnancy.

day 1 following acute MI had no impact on mortality at 1 month in ISIS-4[335] or GISSI-3.[336]

Comments: Not routinely recommended after successful reperfusion or revascularization. Patients receiving IV nitroglycerin should not be switched to oral/transdermal therapy until they have been free from ischemia for 12-24 hours. A nitrate-free interval of at least 10-12 hours is required with oral/transdermal therapy to maintain anti-ischemic effects. All ACS patients should receive sublingual nitroglycerin prior to discharge and instructions for use.

Nitroprusside

Indications and Dose:[248] Hypertensive emergencies; acute heart failure; afterload reduction for acute mitral or aortic regurgitation: IV infusion of 0.3-0.5 mcg/kg/min, titrated every 3-5 minutes to desired effect (usual dose 0.5-8.0 mcg/kg/min). Use lowest effective dose. Maximum dose of 10 mcg/kg/min IV should not be used for longer than 10 minutes. Taper gradually upon discontinuation.

Comments: Nitroprusside improves cardiac output in heart failure primarily through vasodilation (afterload reduction), but it can also decrease ischemia by reducing myocardial work and improving diastolic relaxation. Adverse effects include headache, nausea, vomiting, abdominal discomfort. Nitroprusside can worsen V/Q mismatch and cause hypoxemia in COPD patients who rely on hypoxic pulmonary vasoconstriction to maintain oxygenation. Excessive administration can cause hypotension, tachycardia, myocardial ischemia. Thiocyanate toxicity (tinnitus, blurred vision, mental status changes, abdominal pain, seizures) is uncommon, but is more likely to occur with higher (> 2 mcg/kg/min) doses, prolonged (> 2 day) infusions, or renal failure. Thiocyanate levels should be monitored in these cases; levels < 10 mg/100 mL are usually considered safe. Cyanide toxicity is treated with 3% sodium nitrite followed immediately by sodium thiosulfate. Protect drug reservoir and tubing from light with aluminum foil to avoid deterioration. Use with infusion pump. Hemodynamic monitoring is required to avoid excessive hypotension.

Oxygen

Indications: Often given by convention for ACS, but there are no clear data to support its routine use. Supplemental oxygen is best reserved for patients with respiratory distress or hypoxemia to maintain SaO_2 > 90%.

Comments: Can increase vascular resistance. Can induce hypoventilation and respiratory acidosis in patients with COPD who rely on hypoxic drive for ventilation.

Procainamide

Indications and Dose:[248] Cardiac arrest due to VF or pulseless VT: 20 mg/min IV infusion up to maximum of 17 mg/kg.

Dosages assume normal renal and hepatic function, unless otherwise specified. Check other drug references for complete prescribing information, including dosage adjustments, drug interactions, adverse effects, and safety in pregnancy.

For refractory VF or VT, 100-mg IV bolus doses repeated every 5 minutes can be used. For other indications (stable wide QRS complex tachycardia, SVT resistant to adenosine and vagal maneuvers, rate control of atrial fibrillation in WPW syndrome): 20 mg/min IV infusion until the arrhythmia is suppressed, hypotension develops, QRS widens by 50%, or a total dose of 17 mg/kg is given, followed by an IV maintenance infusion of 1-4 mg/min.

Contraindications: Avoid in patients with a prolonged QT interval or torsade de pointes. Use with caution in conjunction with other drugs that prolong the QT interval.

Comments: Can induce torsade de pointes, especially in patients with renal insufficiency, hypokalemia, or hypomagnesemia. For patients with heart failure or renal insufficiency, the loading dose should be reduced to 12 mg/kg and the maintenance dose reduced to 1-2 mg/min. Blood pressure and ECG should be monitored continuously during IV administration, as sharp drops in blood pressure can occur with rapid infusion, especially in patients with LV dysfunction. Follow blood levels in renal failure and during prolonged use (> 3 mg/min x 24 hours).

Statins (HMG CoA Reductase Inhibitors)

Indications: All ACS patients.
Clinical Trials: Statins reduced early recurrent ischemia when initiated during hospitalization for non-ST-elevation ACS in MIRACL (p. 92).[203] Statins improve long-term event-free survival in patients with coronary artery disease, even if cholesterol levels are within "normal" range.[202] Trials are underway to evaluate the use of statins immediately on presentation vs. after 6 weeks.

Comments: Clinical benefits occur long before changes in plaque morphology, suggesting salutary effects beyond cholesterol lowering and plaque regression.

Warfarin

Indications and Dose: LV thrombus or chronic risk of thromboembolic complications (e.g., atrial fibrillation, prolonged immobilization, low cardiac output): Initial dose of 2.5-10 mg PO daily x 2-4 days, then titrated to maintain an INR of 2.0-3.0. Lower doses may be required in the elderly. Dosage needs to be individualized.

Contraindications: Active bleeding; when risk of bleeding exceeds the benefit of anticoagulation; pregnancy; surgery of CNS or eye; malignant hypertension; lack of patient cooperation. Use with caution in renal or hepatic dysfunction.

Clinical Trials: Long-term anticoagulation with warfarin reduced the risk of recurrent MI or death in ACS patients not receiving aspirin.[388] However, in trials of warfarin vs. aspirin, warfarin resulted in more bleeding complications[389] without reducing reocclusion after successful fibrinolysis[390]

Dosages assume normal renal and hepatic function, unless otherwise specified. Check other drug references for complete prescribing information, including dosage adjustments, drug interactions, adverse effects, and safety in pregnancy.

or death. Recent ACS trials (OASIS-2, CARS, CHAMP) failed to show benefit for the combination of low-intensity warfarin plus aspirin vs. aspirin alone.[391-393] In contrast, studies utilizing higher intensity anticoagulation (INR 2.0-2.5) have demonstrated benefit for aspirin plus warfarin compared to aspirin alone, including 25-50% reductions in death, MI, or stroke in ASPECT-2[394] and WARIS-2,[395] and less reocclusion after fibrinolysis in APRICOT-2.[396]

Comments: Warfarin inhibits synthesis of vitamin K-dependent clotting factors (II, VII, IX, X) and proteins C and S.

Warfarin has no direct effect on existing thrombus but can prevent propagation and embolism of clot. Numerous factors including travel, environment, physical state, and medications can influence the response to therapy. Warfarin interacts with many drugs; check tertiary source for listing. Warfarin's anticoagulant effects can be reversed by vitamin K, fresh whole blood, or fresh frozen plasma (200-500 mL). Studies have shown that systematic follow-up of patients through anticoagulation clinics results in better compliance and control.[397]

Dosages assume normal renal and hepatic function, unless otherwise specified. Check other drug references for complete prescribing information, including dosage adjustments, drug interactions, adverse effects, and safety in pregnancy.

1. Alpert JS, Thygesen K, Antman E, et al. Myocardial infarction redefined—a consensus document of The Joint European Society of Cardiology/American College of Cardiology Committee for the redefinition of myocardial infarction. J Am Coll Cardiol 2000;36:959-69.

1a. Hochman JS, Tamis JE, Thompson TD, et al, for the Global Use of Strategies To Open Occluded Coronary Arteries in Acute Coronary Syndromes IIb Investigators. Sex, clinical presentation, and outcome in patients with acute coronary syndromes. N Engl J Med 1999;341:226-32.

2. Tierney WM, Fitzgerald J, McHenry R. Physician estimates of the probability of myocardial infarction in emergency room patients with chest pain. Med Decis Making 1986;6:12-17.

3. McElroy JB. Angina pectoris with coexisting skeletal chest pain. Am Heart J 1963;66:96-99.

4. Margolis JR, Kannel WS, Feinleib M, et al. Clinical features of unrecognized myocardial infarction—silent and symptomatic. Eighteen year follow-up: the Framingham study. Am J Cardiol 1973;32:1-7.

5. Kannel WB, Abbott RD. Incidence and prognosis of unrecognized myocardial infarction: an update on the Framingham Study. N Engl J Med 1984;311:144-1147.

6. The ECG Criteria Book. Eds: O'Keefe J, Hammill S, Freed M, Pogwizd S. Physicians' Press, Royal Oak, MI, 2002.

7. Fibrinolytic Therapy Trialists' (FTT) Collaborative Group. Indications for fibrinolytic therapy in suspected acute myocardial infarction: collaborative overview of early mortality and major morbidity results from all randomized trials of more than 1000 patients. Lancet 1994; 343:311-322.

8. Barron HV, Bowlby LJ, Breen T, et al. Use of reperfusion therapy for acute myocardial infarction in the United States: data from the National Registry of Myocardial Infarction 2. Circulation 1998;97:1150-6.

9. Matetzky S, Freimark D, Feinberg MS, et al. Acute myocardial infarction with isolated ST-segment elevations revealing acute posterior infarction. J Am Coll Cardiol 1999;34:748-53.

10. Lee TH, Cook EF, Weisberg MC, et al. Impact of the availability of a prior electrocardiogram on the triage of the patient with acute chest pain. J Gen Intern Med 1990;5:381-8.

11. Tsung SH. Several conditions causing elevation of serum CK-MB and CK-BB. Am J Clin Pathol 1981; 75:711-5.

12. Mair J, Morandell D, Genser N, et al. Equivalent early sensitivities of myoglobin, creatine kinase MB mass, creatine kinase isoform ratios, and cardiac troponins I and T for acute myocardial infarction. Clin Chem 1995; 41:1266-72.

13. Puleo PR, Meyer D, Wathen C, et al. Use of a rapid assay of subforms of creatine kinase-MB to diagnose or rule out acute myocardial infarction. N Engl J Med 1994; 331:561-6.

14. Hamm CW, Goldmann BU, Heeschen C, et al. Emergency room triage of patients with acute chest pain by means of rapid testing for cardiac troponin T or troponin I. N Engl J Med 1997; 337:1648-53.

15. Heidenreich PA, Alloggiamento T, Melsop K, et al. The prognostic value of troponin in patients with non-ST-elevation acute coronary syndromes: a meta-analysis. J Am Coll Cardiol 2001; 38:478-85.

16. Morrow DA, Cannon CP, Nader R, et al, for the TACTICS-TIMI 18 Investigators. Ability of minor elevations of troponins I and T to predict benefit from an early invasive strategy in patients with unstable angina and non-ST-elevation myocardial infarction. JAMA 2001;286:2405-2412.

17. Hamm CW, Heeschen C, Goldmann B, et al. Benefit of abciximab in patients with refractory unstable angina in relation to serum troponin levels. N Engl J Med

1999;340:1623-9.

18. Heeschen C, Hamm CW, Goldmann B. Troponin concentrations for stratification of patients with acute coronary syndromes in relation to therapeutic efficacy of tirofiban. Lancet 1999; 354: 1757-62.

19. Ohman EM, Armstrong PW, Christenson RH, for the GUSTO IIA Investigators. Cardiac troponin T levels for risk stratification in acute myocardial ischemia. N Engl J Med 1996; 335:1333-41.

20. Antman EM, Tanasijevic MJ, Thompson B, et al. Cardiac-specific troponin I levels to predict the risk of mortality in patients with acute coronary syndromes. N Engl J Med 1996;335:1342-9.

21. Pettijohn TL, Doyle T, Spiekerman AM, et al. Usefulness of positive troponin-T and negative creatine kinase levels in identifying high-risk patients with unstable angina pectoris. Am J Cardiol 1997;80:510-11.

22. Galvani M, Ottani F, Ferrini D, et al. Prognostic influence of elevated values of cardiac troponin I in patients with unstable angina. Circulation 1997;95:2053-9.

23. Kontos MC, Anderson FP, Schmidt KA, et al. Early diagnosis of acute myocardial infarction in patients without ST-segment elevation. Am J Cardiol 1999;83:155-8.

24. Zaninotto M, Altinier S, Lachin M, et al. Strategies for the early diagnosis of acute myocardial infarction using biochemical markers. Am J Clin Pathol 1999; 111:399-405.

25. Eagle KA, Goodman SG, Avezum A. Practice variation and missed opportunities for reperfusion in ST-segment-elevation myocardial infarction: findings from the Global Registry of Acute Coronary Events (GRACE). Lancet 2002; 359: 373-77.

26. Rogers JR, Canto JG, Lambrew CT, et al. Temporal trends in the treatment of over 1.5 million patients with myocardial infarction in the US from 1990 through 1999. J Am Coll Cardio 2000; 36:2056-63.

27. DeWood MA, Spores J, Notske R, et al. Prevalence of total coronary occlusion during the early hours of transmural myocardial infarction. N Engl J Med 1980;303:897-902.

28. Falk E. Plaque rupture with severe pre-existing stenosis precipitating coronary thrombosis: characteristics of coronary atherosclerotic plaques underlying fatal occlusive thrombi. Br Heart J 1983;50:127-134.

29. Davies MJ, Thomas AC. Plaque fissuring: the cause of acute myocardial infarction, sudden ischaemic death, and crescendo angina. Br Heart J 1985;53:363-373.

30. Rentrop KP, Blanke H, Karsch KR, et al. Acute myocardial infarction: intracoronary application of nitroglycerin and streptokinase. Clin Cardiol 1979;2:354-363.

31. Rentrop P, Blanke H, Karsch KR, et al. Selective intracoronary thrombolysis in acute myocardial infarction and unstable angina pectoris. Circulation 1981;63:307-317.

32. Aversano T, Aversano LT, Passamani E, et al. Atlantic Cardiovascular Patient Outcomes Research Team (C-PORT). Thrombolytic therapy vs primary percutaneous coronary intervention for myocardial infarction in patients presenting to hospitals without on-site cardiac surgery: a randomized controlled trial. JAMA. 2002;287:1943-51.

33. Franzosi MG, Santoro E, De Vita C, et al. Ten-year follow-up of the first megatrial testing thrombolytic therapy in patients with acute myocardial infarction: results of the Gruppo Italiano per lo Studio della Sopravvivenza nell'Infarto-1 study. The GISSI Investigators. Circulation 1998;98:2659-65.

34. Weaver WD, Simes RJ, Ellis SG, et al. Comparison of primary coronary angioplasty and intravenous thrombolytic therapy for acute myocardial infarction. A quantitative review. JAMA 1997;278:2093-2098.

35. Zijlstra F, Jan de Boaer M, Hoorntje JCA, et al. A comparison of immediate coronary angioplasty with intravenous streptokinase in acute myocardial infarction. N Engl J Med 1993;328:680-684.

36. Grines CL, Browne KF, Marco J, et al. A comparison of immediate angioplasty with thrombolytic therapy for acute myocardial infarction. N Engl J Med 1993;328:673-679.

37. Gibbons RJ, Holmes DR, Reeder GS, et al. Immediate angioplasty compared with the administration of a thrombolytic agent followed by conservative treatment for myocardial infarction. N Engl J Med 1993;328:685-691.

38. O'Neill WW, Timmis GC, Bourdillon PD, et al. A prospective randomized clinical trial of intracoronary streptokinase versus coronary angioplasty for acute myocardial infarction. N Engl J Med 1986;341:812-818.

39. DeWood MA, Fisher MJ, for the Spokane Heart Research Group. Direct PTCA versus intravenous rtPA in acute myocardial infarction: preliminary results from a prospective randomized trial. Circulation 1989;80:II-418.

40. Ribeiro EE, Silva LA, Carneiro R, et al. Randomized trial of direct coronary angioplasty versus intravenous streptokinase in acute myocardial infarction. J Am Coll Cardiol 1993;22:376-380.

41. Elizaga J, Garcia EJ, Delcan JL, et al. Primary coronary angioplasty versus systemic thrombolysis in acute anterior myocardial infarction: in-hospital results from a prospective randomized trial. Circulation 1993;88:I-411.

42. Michels KB, Yusuf S. Does PTCA in acute myocardial infarction affect mortality and reinfarction rates? A quantitative overview (meta-analysis) of the randomized clinical trials. Circulation 1995;91:476-485.

43. Zijlstra F, Patel A, Jones M, et al. Clinical characteristics and outcome of patients with early (< 2 h), intermediate (2-4 h) and late (> 4 h) presentation treated by primary coronary angioplasty or thrombolytic therapy for acute myocardial infarction. Eur Heart J 2002;23:550-7.

44. Magid DJ, Calonge BN, Rumsfeld JS, et al. Relation between hospital primary angioplasty volume and mortality for patients with acute MI treated with primary angioplasty vs. thrombolytic therapy. JAMA 2000;284:3131-3138.

45. Amadeo B, Masotti M. Optimal reperfusion in evolving myocardial infarction. Does abciximab improve outcomes in stent treated patients? 2002;39(Supp B):7B.

46. Stone GW, Grines CL, Cox DA, et al. Comparison of angioplasty with stenting, with or without abciximab, in acute myocardial infarction. N Engl J Med, 2002;346:957-66.

47. Andersen HR. Danish trial in acute myocardial infarction (DANAMI) 2. Presented at: American College of Cardiology Scientific Sessions, Atlanta, GA, March, 2002.

48. Grines CL, Westerhausen DR Jr, Grines LL, et al., for the Air PAMI Study Group. A randomized trial of transfer for primary angioplasty versus on-site thrombolysis in patients with high-risk myocardial infarction: the Air-Primary Angioplasty in Myocardial Infarction study. J Am Coll Cardiol 2002; 39:1713-9.

49. Widimsky P, Groch L, Zelizko M, et al. Multicentre randomized trial comparing transport to primary angioplasty vs. immediate thrombolysis vs. combined strategy for patients with acute myocardial infarction presenting to a community hospital without a catheterization laboratory: the PRAGUE study. Eur Heart J 2000;21:823-831.

49a. Widminsky P. PRAGUE-2 study. Presented at the European Society of Cardiology meeting, Berlin, Germany, Sept. 2002.

50. Oldridge NB, Guyatt GH, Fischer ME, et

al. Cardiac rehabilitation after myocardial infarction: combined experience of randomized clinical trials. JAMA 1988;260:945-50.

51. O'Connor GT, Burning JE, Yusuf S, et al. An overview of randomized trials of rehabilitation with exercise after myocardial infarction. Circulation 1989;80:234-44.

52. Kris-Etherton P, Eckel RH, Howard BV, et al. Lyon diet heart study. Benefits of a Mediterranean-style, National Cholesterol Education Program/American Heart Association Step I dietary pattern on cardiovascular disease. Circulation 2001;103:1823-1825.

53. Mori TA, Beilin LJ, Burke V, et al. Interactions between dietary fat, fish, and fish oils and their effects on platelet function in men at risk of cardiovascular disease. Arterioscler Thromb Vasc Biol 1997;17:279-286.

54. Krumholtz HM, Cohen BJ, Tsevat J, et al. Cost-effectiveness of a smoking cessation program after myocardial infarction. J Am Coll Cardiol 1993;22:1697-702.

55. Hambrecht R, Neibauer J, Marburger C, et al. Various intensities of leisure time physical activity in patients with coronary artery disease: effects on cardiorespiratory fitness and progression of coronary atherosclerotic lesions. J Am Coll Cardiol 1993;22:468-77.

56. The Sixth Report of the Joint National Committee on Detection, Evaluation, and Treatment of High Blood Pressure (JNC VI). Arch Intern Med 1997; 157:2413-46.

57. Executive Summary of the Third Report of the National Cholesterol Education Program (NCEP) expert panel on detection, evaluation, and treatment of high blood cholesterol in adults (Adult Treatment Panel III). JAMA 2001;285:2486-97.

58. American Diabetes Association. Standards of medical care for patients with diabetes mellitus. Diabetes Care 2000;23(Suppl l):S32-S42.

59. Antiplatelet Trialists' Collaboration. Secondary prevention of vascular disease by prolonged antiplatelet treatment. Br Med J (Clin Res Ed) 1988;296:320-31.

60. Antiplatelet Trialists' Collaboration. Collaborative overview of randomized trials of antiplatelet therapy, I: prevention of death, myocardial infarction, and stroke by prolonged antiplatelet therapy in various categories of patients. BMJ 1994;308:81-106.

61. Timolol-induced reduction in mortality and reinfarction in patients surviving acute myocardial infarction. N Engl J Med 1981;304:801-7.

62. Randomised trial of cholesterol lowering in 4444 patients with coronary heart disease: the Scandinavian Simvastatin Survival Study (4S). Lancet 1994; 344:1383-9.

63. The Heart Outcomes Prevention Evaluation Study Investigators. Effects of an angiotensin-coverting-enzyme inhibitor, ramipril, on cardiovascular events in high-risk patients. N Engl J Med 2000;342:145-53.

64. Smith SC, Blair SN, Bonow RO, et al. AHA/ACC guidelines for preventing heart attack and death in patients with atherosclerotic cardiovascular disease: 2001 update; a statement for health care professionals from the American Heart Association and the American College of Cardiology. J Am Coll Cardiol 2001;38:1581-3.

65. Ledford SC, Grines CL, Stone GW, et al., for the Primary Angioplasty in Myocardial Infarction (PAMI) Group. Long-term outcome in patients undergoing primary percutaneous intervention: a pooled analysis of the Primary Angioplasty in Myocardial Infarction trials. J Am Coll Cardiol 2002;39(Suppl A);309A.

66. Grines C L, Cox D A, Stone G W, et al. Coronary angioplasty with or without stent implantation for acute myocardial infarction. N Engl J Med 1999;341:1949-56.

66a. Kandzari DE, Hasselblad V, Tcheng JE, et al. Improved clinical outcomes with abciximab therapy in acute myocardial infarction: A systematic overview of randomized clinical trials. Accepted for presentation at ACC 2003.

67. Ross AM, Coyne KS, Reiner JS, et al. A randomized trial comparing primary angioplasty with a strategy of short acting thrombolysis and immediate planned rescue angioplasty in acute myocardial infarction: the PACT trial. J Am Coll Cardiol 1999;34:1954-1962.

68. Berkowitz SD, Sane DC, Sigmon KN, et al. Occurrence and clinical significance of thrombocytopenia in a population undergoing high-risk percutaneous coronary revascularization. J Am Coll Cardiol 1998;32:311-9.

69. Montalescot G, Barragan P, Wittenberg O, et al. Platelet glycoprotein IIb/IIIa inhibition with coronary stenting for acute myocardial infarction. N Engl J Med 2001;344:1895-903.

70. Kastrati A, Mehilli J, Dirschinger J, et al. Myocardial salvage after coronary stenting plus abciximab versus fibrinolysis plus abciximab in patients with acute myocardial infarction: a randomized trial. Lancet 2002;359:920-25.

71. Maillard L, Hamon M, Khalife K, et al. A comparison of systematic stenting and conventional balloon angioplasty during primary percutaneous transluminal coronary angioplasty for acute myocardial infarction. J Am Coll Cardiol 2000;35:1729 –36.

72. Antoniucci D, Santoro G M, Bolognese L, et al. A clinical trial comparing primary stenting of the infarct-related artery with optimal primary angioplasty of acute myocardial infarction. Results from the Florence Randomized Elective Stenting in Acute Coronary Occlusions (FRESCO) trial. J Am Coll Cardiol 1998;3:1234- 9.

73. Saito S, Hosokawa G, Tanaka S, Nakamura S. Primary stent implantation is superior to balloon angioplasty in acute myocardial infarction: final results the primary angioplasty versus stent implantation in acute myocardial infarction (PASTA) trial. Cathet Cardiovasc Intervent 1999;48:262-8.

74. Lansky AJ, Stone GW. Percutaneous intervention for acute coronary syndromes. Eds: Safian, RD, Freed, MS. In: The Manual of Interventional Cardiology, 3rd Edition. Physicians' Press, Royal Oak, MI, 2001.

75. Lee L, Erbel R, Brown TM, et al. Multicenter registry of angioplasty therapy of cardiogenic shock: initial and long-term survival. J Am Coll Cardiol 1991;17:599-603.

76. O'Neill WW, Erbel R, Laufer N, et al. Coronary angioplasty therapy of cardiogenic shock complicating acute myocardial infarction. Circulation 1995;72:III-309.

77. Hochman JS, Boland J, Sleeper LA, et al., and the SHOCK Registry Investigators. Current spectrum of cardiogenic shock and effect of early revascularization on mortality. Circulation 1995;91:372-88.

78. Holmes DR, Bates EF, Kleiman NS, et al. Contemporary reperfusion therapy for cardiogenic shock: the GUSTO-I trial experience. J Am Coll Cardiol 1995;26:668-674.

79. Disler L, Haitas B, Benjamin J, et al. Cardiogenic shock in evolving myocardial infarction: treatment by angioplasty and streptokinase. Heart Lung 1987;16:649.

80. Hochman JS, Sleeper LA, White HW, et al. One-year survival following early revascularization for cardiogenic shock. JAMA 2001;285:190-192.

81. Morice MC, Serruys PW, Sousa E, et al. A randomized comparison of a sirolimus-eluting stent with a standard stent for coronary revascularization. N Engl J Med 2002;346:1773-80.

82. Goodman, S. Presented at PCR meeting, Paris, France, May, 2002.

83. Presented at PCR meeting, Paris, France, May, 2002.

84. Grube E, Lansky AJ, Reifart N, et al. SCORE six-month angiographic results: Improved restenosis in patients receiving the QUADDS-QP2 drug-eluting stent compared with the control, bare stents. J Am Coll Cardiol 2002;39 (suppl. A):59A.

85. Berger PB, Steinhubl S. Clinical implications of percutaneous coronary intervention–clopidogrel in unstable angina to prevent recurrent events (PCI-CURE) study: A US perspective. Circulation 2002;106:2284-7.

86. Armstrong PW, Collen D. Fibrinolysis for acute myocardial infarction. Circulation 2001;103:2862-2866.

87. The GUSTO investigators. An international randomized trial comparing four thrombolytic strategies for acute myocardial infarction. N Engl J Med 1993;329:673-682.

88. ASSENT-2 Investigators. Single-bolus tenecteplase compared with front-loaded alteplase in acute myocardial infarction: the ASSENT-2 double blind randomized trial. Lancet 1999;354:716-722.

89. GUSTO III Investigators. A comparison of reteplase with alteplase for acute myocardial infarction. N Engl J Med. 1997;337:1124-1130.

90. Topol E, Ohman EM, Armstrong PW, et al., for the GUSTO III Investigators. Survival outcomes one year after reperfusion therapy with either alteplase or reteplase for AMI: results from GUSTO III trial. Circulation 2000; 102:1761-1765.

91. Ryan TJ, Anderson JL, Antman EM, Braniff BA, Brooks NH, Califf RM, Hillis LD, Hiratzka LF, Rapaport E, Riegel BJ, Russell RO, Smith EE III, Weaver WD. ACC/AHA guidelines for the management of patients with acute myocardial infarction: a report of the American College of Cardiology/American Heart Association Task Force on Practice Guidelines (Committee on Management of Acute

Myocardial Infarction). J Am Coll Cardiol 1996;28:1328-1428.

92. Ryan TJ, Antman EM, Brooks NH, Califf RM, Hillis LD, Hiratzka LF, Rapaport E, Riegel B, Russell RO, Smith EE III, Weaver WD. 1999 update: ACC/AHA guidelines for the management of patients with acute myocardial infarction: a report of the American College of Cardiology/American Heart Association Task Force on Practice Guidelines (Committee on Management of Acute Myocardial Infarction). J Am Coll Cardiol 1999;34:890-911.

93. The Hirulog and Early Reperfusion or Occlusion (HERO)-2 Trial Investigators. Thrombin-specific anticoagulation with bivalirudin versus heparin in patients receiving fibrinolytic therapy for acute myocardial infarction: the HERO-2 randomized trial. Lancet 2001; 358:1855-63.

94. The Assessment of the Safety and Efficacy of a New Thrombolytic Regimen (ASSENT)-3 Investigators. Efficacy and safety of tenecteplase in combination with enoxaparin, abciximab, or unfractionated heparin: the ASSENT-3 randomized trial in acute myocardial infarction. Lancet 2001;358:605-13.

95. Ross AM, Reiner JS, Thompson MA, et al. Immediate and follow-up procedural outcome of 214 patients undergoing rescue PTCA in the GUSTO trial: no effect of the lytic agent. Circulation 1993;88(Suppl I):I-410(abstr).

96. Ellis SG, Ribeiro da Silva E, Heyndrickx G, et al. Randomized comparison of rescue angioplasty with conservative management of patients with early failure of thrombolysis for acute anterior myocardial infarction. Circulation 1994;90:2280-2284.

97. The CORAMI Study Group. Outcome of attempted rescue coronary angioplasty after failed thrombolysis for acute myocardial infarction. Am J Cardiol 1994;74:172-174.

98. Miller JM, Smalling R, Ohman EM, Bode

C, Betriu A, Kleiman NS, Schildcrout JS, Bastos E, Topol EJ, Califf RM. Effectiveness of early coronary angioplasty and abciximab for failed thrombolysis (reteplase or alteplase) during acute myocardial infarction (results from the GUSTO-III trial). Global Use of Strategies To Open occluded coronary arteries. Am J Cardiol 1999;84:779-84.

99. McKendall et al. J Am Coll Cardiol 1997;29:389A.

100. Gibson CM, Cannon CP, Piana RN, et al. Rescue PTCA in the TIMI 4 trial. J Am Coll Cardiol 1994;1A-48A:225A.

101. Wnqk A, Krupa H, Gasior M, et al. Results of rescue-angioplasty after unsuccessful intracoronary streptokinase therapy in patients with acute myocardial infarction. European Congress of Cardiology, abstract, 1995.

102. Adamian MG, Stone GW, Mehran R, et al. Have the outcomes of rescue angioplasty after failed thrombolytic therapy in acute myocardial infarction improved in the stent era? J Am Coll Cardiol. 2002;39(Suppl A):309A.

103. Rogers WJ, Baim DS, Fore JM, et al for the TIMI-IIA investigators. Comparison of immediate invasive, delayed invasive, and conservative strategies after tissue-type plasminogen activator. Circulation 1990;81:1457-1476.

104. Topol EJ, Califf RM, George BS, et al., and the Thrombolysis and Angioplasty in Myocardial Infarction Study Group. A randomized trial of immediate versus delayed elective angioplasty after intravenous tissue plasminogen activator in acute myocardial infarction. N Engl J Med 1987;317:581-588.

105. Simoons ML, Arnold AET, Bertriu A, et al. Thrombolysis with tissue plasminogen activator in acute myocardial infarction: no additional benefit from immediate percutaneous coronary angioplasty. Lancet 1988;1:197-202.

106. Gibson C, Cannon C, Piana R. Angiographic predictors of reocclusion after thrombolysis: Results from the Thrombolysis In Myocardial Infarction (TIMI-4) trial. J Am Coll Cardiol 1995;25:589-9.

107. The TIMI Study Group. Comparison of invasive and conservative strategies after treatment with intravenous tissue plasminogen activator in acute myocardial infarction. Results of the Thrombolysis in Myocardial Infarction (TIMI) phase II trial. N Engl J Med 1989;320:618-27.

108. Topol EJ, Califf RM, Vandormael M, et al., and the Thrombolysis and Angioplasty in Myocardial Infarction-6 Study Group. A randomized trial of late reperfusion therapy for acute myocardial infarction. Circulation 1992;85:2090-2099.

109. Van de Werf F. Discrepancies between the effects of coronary reperfusion on survival and left ventricular function. Lancet 1989;I:1367-1369.

110. Galvani M, Ottani F, Ferrini D, et al. Patency of the infarct-related artery and left ventricular function as the major determinants of survival after Q-wave acute myocardial infarction. Am J Cardiol 1993;71:1-7.

111. Anderson JL. Overview of patency as an endpoint of thrombolytic therapy. Am J Cardiol 1991;67:11-16E.

112. Madsen J, Grande P, et al. Danish multi-center randomized study of invasive versus conservative treatment in patients with inducible ischemia after thrombolysis in acute myocardial infarction (DANAMI). Circulation 1997;96:748-755.

113. ISIS-3 (Third International Study of Infarct Survival) Collaborative Group. A randomized comparison of streptokinase vs. tissue plasminogen activator vs. anistreplase and of aspirin plus heparin vs. aspirin alone among 4,1 299 cases of suspected acute myocardial infarction: ISIS-3. Lancet 1992;339:753-770.

114. Maggioni AP, Franzosi MG, Santoro E, et al. The risk of stroke in patients with acute myocardial infarction after thrombolytic and antithrombotic treatment. Gruppo italiano per lo Studio della Sopravvivenza nell'Infarto Miocardico II (GISSI-2), and The International Study Group. N Engl J Med 1992;327:1-6.

115. Topol EJ, Ohman EM, Armstrong PW, et al. Survival outcomes 1 year after reperfusion therapy with either alteplase or reteplase for acute myocardial infarction: results from the Global Utilization of Streptokinase and t-PA for Occluded Coronary Arteries (GUSTO) III Trial. Circulation 2000;102:1761-5.

116. Ito H, Okamura A, Iwakura K, et al. Myocardial perfusion patterns related to thrombolysis in myocardial infarction perfusion grades after coronary angioplasty in patients with acute anterior wall myocardial infarction. Circulation. 1996;93:1993-1999.

117. Kleiman N, Ohman E, et al. Profound inhibition of platelet aggregation with monoclonal antibody 7E3Fab after thrombolytic therapy: results from the Thrombolysis and Angioplasty in myocardial infarction (TAMI) 8 pilot study. J Am Coll Cardiol 1993;22:381-389.

118. Ohman E, Kleiman N, et al. Combined accelerated tissue plasminogen activator and platelet glycoprotein IIb/IIIa integrin receptor blockade in acute myocardial infarction: results of a randomized placebo controlled dose ranging trial. Circulation 1997:95:846-854.

119. The PARADIGM Investigators. Combined thrombolysis with the platelet glycoprotein IIb/IIIa inhibitor lamifiban: results of the platelet aggregation receptor antagonist dose investigation and reperfusion gain in myocardial infarction (PARADIGM) trial. J Am Coll Cardiol 1998;32:2003-2010.

120. Antman EM, Gibson CM, de Lemos JA, et al. Combination reperfusion therapy with abciximab and reduced dose reteplase: results from TIMI 14. The Thrombolysis in Myocardial Infarction (TIMI) 14 Investigators. Eur Heart J. 2000;21:1944-53.

121. Herrmann HC, Moliterno DJ, Ohman EM, et al. Facilitation of early percutaneous coronary intervention after reteplase with or without abciximab in acute myocardial infarction: results from the SPEED (GUSTO-4 Pilot) trial. J Am Coll Cardiol 2000;36:1489-96.

122. The Assessment of the Safety and Efficacy of a New Thrombolytic Regimen (ASSENT)-3 Investigators. Efficacy and safety of tenecteplase in combination with enoxaparin, abciximab, or unfractionated heparin: the ASSENT-3 randomized trial in acute myocardial infarction. Lancet 2001;358:605-13.

123. The GUSTO V Investigators. Reperfusion therapy for acute myocardial infarction with fibrinolytic therapy or combination reduced fibrinolytic therapy and platelet glycoprotein IIb/IIIa inhibition: the GUSTO V randomized trial. Lancet 2001;357:1905-14.

124. Braunwald E. Unstable angina classification. Circulation 1989;80:410-4.

125. Slater DK, Hlatky MA, Mark DB, et al. Outcome in suspected acute myocardial infarction with normal or minimally abnormal admission electrocardiographic findings. Am J Cardiol 1987;60:766-70.

126. de Zwaan C, Bar FW, Janssen JH, et al. Angiographic and clinical characteristics of patients with unstable angina showing an ECG pattern indicating critical narrowing of the proximal LAD coronary artery. Am Heart J 1989;117:657-65.

127. Cannon CP, McCabe CH, Stone PH, et al. The electrocardiogram predicts one-year outcome of patients with unstable angina and non-Q wave myocardial infarction: results of the TIMI III registry

ECG ancillary study. J Am Coll Cardiol 1997;30:133-140.

128. Ryan TJ, Anderson JL, Antman EM, Braniff BA, Brooks NH, Califf RM, Hillis LD, Hiratzka LF, Rapaport E, Riegel BJ, Russell RO, Smith EE III, Weaver WD. ACC/AHA guidelines for the management of patients with acute myocardial infarction: a report of the American College of Cardiology/American Heart Association Task Force on Practice Guidelines (Committee on Management of Acute Myocardial Infarction). J Am Coll Cardiol 1996;28:1328-1428.

129. Roberts R, Fromm RE. Management of acute coronary syndromes based on risk stratification by biochemical markers: an idea whose time has come. Circulation 1998;98:1831-3.

130. Morrow DA, Rifai N, Antman EM, et al. C-reactive protein is a potent predictor of mortality independently of and in combination with troponin T in acute coronary syndromes: a TIMI 11A substudy. J Am Coll Cardiol 1998;31:1460-1465.

131. Biasucci LM, Liuzzo G, Grillo RL, et al. Elevated levels of C-reactive protein at discharge in patients with unstable angina predict recurrent instability. Circulation 1999;99:855-860.

132. Lindmark E, Diderholm E, Wallentin L, et al. Relationship between interleukin 6 and mortality in patients with unstable coronary artery disease: effects of an early invasive or noninvasive strategy. JAMA 286;2107-2113.

133. Cheitlin ME, Hutter AM, Brindis RG, et al. Use of sildenafil (Viagra) in patients with cardiovascular disease. AHA/ACC expert consensus document. J Am Coll Cardiol 1999;33:273-82.

134. Report of The Holland Interuniversity Nifedipine/Metoprolol Trial (HINT) Research Group. Early treatment of unstable angina in the coronary care unit: a randomized, double blind, placebo controlled comparison of recurrent ischemia in patients treated with nifedipine or metoprolol or both. Br Heart J 1986;56:400-13.

135. The TIMI IIIB Trial Investigators. Effects of tissue plasminogen activator and a comparison of early invasive and conservative strategies in unstable angina and non-Q-wave myocardial infarction. Results of the TIMI IIIB trial. Circulation 1994;89:1545-56.

136. The EPISTENT Investigators. Randomized placebo-controlled and balloon-angioplasty-controlled trial to assess safety of coronary stenting with use of platelet glycoprotein IIb/IIIa blockade. Lancet 1998;352:87-92.

137. The CAPTURE Investigators. Randomized placebo-controlled trial of abciximab before and during coronary intervention in refractory unstable angina: the CAPTURE study. Lancet 1997;349:2429-35.

138. O'Shea JC, Buller CE, Cantor WJ, et al. Long-term efficacy of platelet glycoprotein IIb/IIIa integrin blockade with eptifibatide in coronary stent intervention. JAMA 2002;287:618-621.

139. The IMPACT-II Investigators. Randomized placebo-controlled trial of effect of eptifibatide on complications of percutaneous coronary intervention: IMPACT-II. Lancet 1997;349:1422-28.

140. The PURSUIT Trial Investigators. Inhibition of platelet glycoprotein IIb/IIIa with eptifibatide in patients with acute coronary syndromes. N Eng J Med 1998;339:436-43.

141. The RESTORE Investigators. Effects of platelet glycoprotein IIb/IIIa blockade with tirofiban on adverse cardiac event in patients with unstable angina or acute myocardial infarction undergoing coronary angioplasty. Circulation 1997; 96:1445-53.

142. Gibson CM, Goel M, Cohen DJ, et al.

Six-month angiographic and clinical follow-up of patients prospectively randomized to receive either tirofiban or placebo during angioplasty in the RESTORE trial. J Am Coll Cardiol 1998;32:28-34.

143. Cannon CP, Weintraub WS, Demopoulos LA, et al. Comparison of early invasive and conservative strategies in patients with unstable coronary syndromes treated with the glycoprotein IIb/IIIa inhibitor tirofiban. N Engl J Med 2001;344:1879-87.

144. Stone GW, Moliterno DJ, Bertrand M, et al. Impact of clinical syndrome acuity on the differential response to 2 glycoprotein IIb/IIIa inhibitors in patients undergoing coronary stenting: the TARGET Trial. Circulation 2002;105:2347-54.

145. Gibbons RJ, Chatterjee K, Daley J, et al. ACC/AHA/ACP-ASIM guidelines for the management of patients with chronic stable angina. J Am Coll Cardiol 1999;33:2092-197.

146. TIMI-3B Investigators. Effects of tissue plasminogen activator and a comparison of early invasive and conservative strategies in unstable angina and non Q-wave myocardial infarction. Circulation 1994;89:1545-1556.

147. Boden W. O'Rourke R, et al. Outcomes in patients with acute non-Q-wave myocardial infarction randomly assigned to an invasive as compared with a conservative management strategy. N Engl J Med 1998;338:1785-92.

148. Fragmin and Fast Revascularization during Instability in Coronary artery disease (FRISC II) Investigators. Long-term low-molecular-mass heparin in unstable coronary-artery disease: FRISC II prospective randomized multicenter study. Lancet 1999; 354:701-7.

148a. Fox KA, Poole-Wilson PA, Henderson RA, et al. Interventional versus conservative treatment for patients with unstable angina or non-ST-elevation myocardial infarction: the British Heart Foundation RITA 3 randomized trial. Published in Lancet on-line, September 1, 2002, http://image.thelancet.com/extras/02art8090web.pdf.

148b. Lagerqvist B, Husted S, Kontny F, et al. Long-term perspective on the protective effects of an early invasive strategy in unstable coronary disease. Two-year follow-up of the FRISC-II invasive study. J Am Coll Cardiol 2002;40:1902-1914.

149. Singh M, Holmes DR, Garratt KN, et al. Stents versus conventional PTCA in unstable angina. J Am Coll Cardiol 1999;33-29A.

149a. Glaser R, Herrmann, HC, Murphy, SA, et al. Benefit of an early invasive management strategy in women with acute coronary syndromes. JAMA 2002;288:3124-9.

150. Topol EJ, Mark DB, Lincoff AM, et al. Outcomes at 1 year and economic implications of platelet glycoprotein IIb/IIIa blockade in patients undergoing coronary stenting: results from a multicenter randomized trial. EPISTENT Investigators. Evaluation of platelet IIb/IIIa inhibitor for stenting. Lancet 1999 ;354:2019-24.

151. PRISM-PLUS Study Investigators. Inhibition of the platelet glycoprotein IIb/IIIa receptor with tirofiban in unstable angina and non-Q-wave myocardial infarction. N Engl J Med 1998;338:1488-97.

152. Fourth American College of Chest Physicians Consensus Conference on Antithrombotic Therapy. Chest. 1995;108(suppl):225S-522S.

153. Schwartz L, Bourassa MG, Lesperance J, et al. Aspirin and dipyridamole in the prevention of restenosis after percutaneous transluminal coronary angioplasty. N Engl J Med 1988;318:1714-1719.

154. Mufson L, Black A, Roubin G, et al. A randomized trial of aspirin in PTCA:

effect of high vs. low dose aspirin on major complications and restenosis. J Am Coll Cardiol 1988;11:236A.

155. Henderson W, Goldman S, Copeland J, et al. Antiplatelet or anticoagulant therapy after coronary artery bypass surgery: a meta-analysis of clinical trials. Ann Intern Med 1989;111:743-750.

156. White CW, Chaitman B, Knudtson ML, et al. Antiplatelet agents are effective in reducing the acute ischemic complications of angioplasty but do not prevent restenosis: results from the ticlopidine trial. Coronary Artery Dis 1991;2:757.

157. Gum PA, Kottke-Marchant K, Poggio ED, et al. Profile and prevalence of aspirin resistance among patients with heart disease: a prospective, comprehensive assessment. Circulation 2000;18:II-418.

158. Schrör K. The basic pharmacology of ticlopidine and clopidogrel. Platelets 1993;4:252-61.

159. Savi P, Heilmann E, Nurden P, et al. Clopidogrel: an antithrombic drug acting on the ADP-dependant activation pathway of human platelets. Clin Appl Thromb/Hemost 1996;2:35-42.

160. Boneu B, Destelle G. Platelet anti-aggregating activity and tolerance of clopidogrel in atherosclerotic patients. Thromb Haemost 1996;76:939-43.

161. CAPRIE steering committee. A randomized blinded trial of clopidogrel versus aspirin in patients at risk of ischemic events. Lancet 1996;348:1329-39.

162. Yusuf S, Zhao F, Mehta SR, et al. Effects of clopidogrel in addition to aspirin in patients with acute coronary syndromes without ST-segment elevation. N Engl J Med 2001;345:494-502.

163. Mehta SR, Yusuf S, Peters RJ, et al. Effects of pretreatment with clopidogrel and aspirin followed by long-term therapy in patients undergoing percutaneous coronary intervention: the PCI-CURE study. Lancet 2001;358:527-33.

164. Bertrand ME, Rupprecht H-J, Urban P, et al., for the CLASSICS Investigators. Double-blind study of the safety of clopidogrel with and without a loading dose in combination with aspirin compared with ticlopidine in combination with aspirin after coronary stenting. The Clopidogrel Aspirin Stent International Cooperative Study (CLASSICS). Circulation 2000;102:642-629.

165. Bhatt D, Topol EJ. Clopidogrel resulted in fewer major adverse cardiac events after stenting compared with ticlopidine. Eur Heart J 2000;21:281.

166. CAPRIE steering committee. A randomized blinded trial of clopidogrel versus aspirin in patients at risk of ischemic events. (CAPRIE) Lancet 1996;348:1329-39.

167. Bennett CL, Connors JM, Carwile JM, et al. Thrombotic thrombocytopenia purpura associated with clopidogrel. N Engl J Med 2000;342(24):1773-7.

168. Bennett CL, Weinberg PD, Rozenberg-Ben-Dror K, et al. Thrombotic thrombocytopenia purpura associated with ticlopidine: a review of 60 cases. Ann Intern Med 1998;128:541-4.

169. Alexander JH, Ohman EM, Harrington RA. Platelet GP IIb/IIIa inhibitors in acute MI: pathophysiology and clinical effects. Acute Coronary Syndromes 1998;1:46-51.

170. Lefkovits J, Plow EF, Topol EJ. Platelet glycoprotein IIb/IIIa receptors in cardiovascular medicine. N Engl J Med 1995;332:1553-9.

170a. Newby LK, Ohman EM, Christenson RH, et al. Benefit of glycoprotein IIb/IIIa inhibition in patients with acute coronary syndromes and troponin T-positive status: the Paragon-B troponin T substudy. Circulation 2001;103:2891-6.

171. Topol EJ, Byzova TV, Plow EF. Platelet GPIIb-IIIa blockers. Lancet 1999;353:227-31.

172. Coller BS. Potential non-glycoprotein IIb/IIIa effects of abciximab. Am Heart J 1999;138:S1-5.

173. Tam SH, Sassoli PM, Jordan RE, Nakada MT. Abciximab (ReoPro, chimeric 7E3 Fab) demonstrates equivalent affinity and functional blockade of glycoprotein IIb/IIIa and $a_v\beta_3$ integrins. Circulation 1998;98:1085-91.

174. Phillips DR., Scarborough RM. Clinical pharmacology of eptifibatide. Am J Cardiol 1997;80:11B-20B.

175. Harrington RA, Kleiman NS, Kottke-Marchant K, et al. Immediate and reversible platelet inhibition after intravenous administration of a peptide glycoprotein IIb/IIIa inhibitor during percutaneous coronary intervention. Am J Cardiol 1995;76:1222-27.

176. Theroux P. Tirofiban. Drugs of Today 1999;35:59-73.

177. The EPIC Investigators. Use of a monoclonal antibody directed against the platelet glycoprotein IIb/IIIa receptor in high-risk coronary angioplasty. N Engl J Med 1994;330:956-961.

178. The EPILOG Investigators. Platelet glycoprotein IIb/IIIa receptor blockade and low-dose heparin during percutaneous coronary revascularization. N Engl J Med 1997;336:1689-1696.

179. Gammie JS, Zenati M, Kormos RL, et al. Abciximab and excessive bleeding in patients undergoing emergency cardiac operations. Ann Thorac Surg 1998;65:465-9.

180. Alvarez JM. Emergency coronary bypass grafting for failed percutaneous coronary artery stenting: increased costs and platelet transfusion requirements after the use of abciximab. J Thorac Cardiovasc Surg 1998;115:472-3.

181. Hirsh J, Anand SS, Halperin JL, et al. Guide to anticoagulant therapy: heparin. A statement for healthcare professionals from the American Heart Association. Circulation 2001;103:2994-3018.

182. Antman EM. The search for replacements for unfractionated heparin. Circulation 2001;103:2310-2314.

183. Fareed J, Hoppensteadt DA, Bick RL. An update on heparins at the beginning of the new millenium. Semin Thromb Hemost 2000;26:5-21.

184. Cannon CP, Antman EM, Crawford MH. Heparin and low-molecular-weight heparin in acute coronary syndromes and angioplasty. In: Crawford MH, editor. Cardiology Clinics: Annual of Drug Therapy. Philadelphia: WB Saunders;1997:105-19.

185. Cohen M, Demers C, Gurfinkel EP, et al, for the Efficacy and Safety of Subcutaneous Enoxaparin in Non-Q-Wave Coronary Events Study Group. A comparison of low-molecular-weight heparin with unfractionated heparin for unstable coronary artery disease. N Engl J Med 1997;337:447-52.

186. Antman EM, McCabe CH, Gurfinkel EP, et al. Enoxaparin prevents death and cardiac ischemic events in unstable angina/non-Q-wave myocardial infarction: results of the Thrombolysis In Myocardial Infarction (TIMI) 11B trial. Circulation 1999;100:1593-601.

187. Antman EM, Cohen M, Radley D, et al. Assessment of the treatment effect of enoxaparin for unstable angina/non-Q-wave myocardial infarction. TIMI 11B-ESSENCE meta-analysis. Circulation 1999;100:1602-8.

188. Antman EM, Cohen M, McCabe C, et al., for the TIMI 11B and ESSENCE Investigators. Enoxaparin is superior to unfractionated heparin for preventing clinical events at 1-year follow-up of TIMI 11B and ESSENCE. Eur Heart J 2002;23:308-14.

189. Klein W, Buchwald A, Hillis SE, et al. Comparison of low-molecular-weight heparin with unfractionated heparin acutely and with placebo for 6 weeks in the management of unstable coronary

artery disease: Fragmin in coronary artery disease study (FRIC). Circulation 1997;96:61-68.

190. The FRAXIS Study Group. Comparison of two treatment durations (6 days and 14 days) of a low molecular weight heparin with a 6-day treatment of unfractionated heparin in the initial management of unstable angina or non-Q-wave myocardial infarction: FRAXIS (Fraxiparine in Ischaemic Syndrome). Eur Heart J 1999;20:1553-1562.

191. Weitz JI. Low-molecular-weight heparins [published erratum appears in N Engl J Med 1997;337:1567]. N Engl J Med 1997;337:688-98.

192. Kereiakes DJ, Grines C, Fry E, et al. Enoxaparin and abciximab adjunctive pharmacotherapy during percutaneous coronary intervention. J Invasive Cardiol 2001;13:272-8.

193. Young JJ, Kereiakes DJ, Grines CL. Low-molecular-weight heparin therapy in percutaneous coronary intervention: the NICE 1 and NICE 4 trials. National Investigators Collaborating on Enoxaparin Investigators. J Invasive Cardiol 2000;12(Suppl E):E14-8; discussion E25-8.

194. Ferguson JJ. Combining low-molecular-weight heparin and glycoprotein IIb/IIIa antagonists for the treatment of acute coronary syndromes: the NICE 3 story. National Investigators Collaborating on Enoxaparin. J Invasive Cardiol 2000;12(Suppl E):E10-3; discussion E25-8.

195. Cohen M. Initial experience with the low-molecular-weight heparin, enoxaparin, in combination with the platelet glycoprotein IIb/IIIa blocker, tirofiban, in patients with non-ST segment elevation acute coronary syndromes. J Invasive Cardiol 2000;12(Suppl E):E5-9; discussion E25-8.

196. Bhatt DL. Presented at the American Heart Association meeting, Anaheim, CA,

November, 2001.

197. Presented at the American College of Cardiology meeting, Atlanta, GA, March, 2002.

198. Lovenox. Physicians' Desk Reference. Medical Economics 2002, 56th edition, p. 750.

199. Lefkovits J, Topol E. Direct thrombin inhibitors in cardiovascular medicine. Circulation 1994;90:1522-1536.

200. The Direct Thrombin Inhibitor Trialists' Collaborative Group. Direct thrombin inhibitors in acute coronary syndromes: principal results of a meta-analysis based on individual patients' data. Lancet 2002; 359:294-302.

201. Greinacher A, Lubenow N. Recombinant hirudin in clinical practice: focus on lepirudin. Circulation 2001;103:1479-1484.

202. Expert Panel on Detection, Evaluation, and Treatment of High Blood Cholesterol in Adults. Executive summary of the third report of the National Cholesterol Education Program (NCEP) expert panel on detection, evaluation and treatment of high blood cholesterol in adults (Adult Treatment Panel III). JAMA 2001;285:2486-97.

203. Schwartz GG, Olsson AG, Ezekowitz MD, et al. Effects of atorvastatin on early recurrent ischemic events in acute coronary syndromes. JAMA 2001;285:1711-1718.

204. Heeschen C, Hamm CW, Laufs U, et al., for the Platelet Receptor Inhibition in Ischemic Syndrome Management (PRISM) Investigators. Withdrawal of statins increases event rates in patients with acute coronary syndromes. Circulation 2002;105:1446-52.

205. Fonarow GC, Gawlinski A, Moughrabi S, et al. Improved treatment of coronary heart disease by implementation of a cardiac hospitalization atherosclerosis management program (CHAMP). Am J Cardiol 2001;87:819-22.

206. Boersma E, Harrington RA, Moliterno DJ, et al. Platelet glycoprotein IIb/IIIa inhibitors in acute coronary syndromes: a meta-analysis of all major randomized clinical trials. Lancet 2002;359:189-98.

207. Robertson RM. Women and cardiovascular disease: the misconception and the need for action. Circulation 2001;103:2318-2320.

208. Hulley S, Grady D, Bush T, et al. Randomized trial of estrogen plus progestin for secondary prevention of coronary heart disease in postmenopausal women. Heart and estrogen/progestin replacement study (HERS) research group. JAMA 1998;280:605-13.

209. Kip KE, Faxon DP, Detre KM, et al. Coronary angioplasty in diabetic patients: the National Heart, Lung, and Blood Institute percutaneous transluminal coronary angioplasty registry. Circulation 1996;94:1818-25.

210. Fava S, Azzopardi J, Agium-Muscat H. Outcome of unstable angina in patients with diabetes mellitus. Diabet Med 1997;14:209-13.

211. The BARI Investigators. Seven-year outcome in the Bypass Angioplasty Revascularization Investigation (BARI) by treatment and diabetic status. J Am Coll Cardiol 2000;35:1122-9.

212. Chen L, Theroux P, Lesperance J, et al. Angiographic features of vein grafts versus ungrafted coronary arteries in patients with unstable angina and previous bypass surgery. J Am Coll Cardiol 1996;28:1493-9.

213. Silva JA, White CJ, Collins TJ, Ramee SR. Morphologic comparison of atherosclerotic lesions in native coronary arteries and saphenous vein grafts with intracoronary angioscopy in patients with unstable angina. Am Heart J 1998;136:156-63.

214. Waters DD, Walling A, Roy D, Theroux P. Previous coronary artery bypass grafting as an adverse prognostic factor in unstable angina pectoris. Am J Cardiol 1986;58:465-9.

215. Kleiman NS, Anderson HV, Rogers WJ, et al. Comparison of outcome of patients with unstable angina and non-Q-wave acute myocardial infarction with and without prior coronary artery bypass grafting (Thrombolysis in Myocardial Ischemia III Registry). Am J Cardiol 1996;77:227-31.

216. Brogan WC, Lange RA, Kim AS, et al. Alleviation of cocaine-induced coronary vasoconstriction by nitroglycerin. J Am Coll Cardiol 1991;18:581-6.

217. Yao SS, Spindola-Franco H, Menegus M, et al. Successful intracoronary thrombolysis in cocaine-induced acute myocardial infarction. Cathet Cardiovasc Diagn 1997;42:294-7.

218. Hollander JE. The management of cocaine-associated myocardial ischemia. N Engl J Med 1995;33:1267-72.

219. Isner JM, Chokshi SK. Cardiovascular complications of cocaine. Curr Probi Cardiol 1991;16:89-123.

220. Isner JM, Chokshi SK. Cocaine and vasospasm. N Engl J Med 1989;321:1604-6.

221. Opie LH. Calcium channel antagonists in the management of anginal syndromes: changing concepts in relation to the role of coronary vasospasm. Prog Cardiovasc Dis 1996;38:291-314.

222. Chahine RA, Feldman RL, Giles TD, et al. Randomized placebo controlled trial of amlodipine in vasospastic angina. J Am Coll Cardiol 1993;21:1365-70.

222a. Greenbaum AB, Harrington RA, Hudson MP, et al. Therapeutic value of eptifibatide at community hospitals transferring patients to tertiary referral centers early after admission for acute coronary syndromes. PURSUIT Investigators. J Am Coll Cardiol 2001;37:492-8.

223. Califf RM, Topol EJ, Stack RS, et al. Evaluation of combination thrombolytic

therapy and timing of cardiac catheterization in acute myocardial infarction. Results of Thrombolysis and Angioplasty in Myocardial Infarction–phase 5 randomized trial. TAMI Study Group. Circulation 1991;83:1543-56.

224. Detre KM, Lombardero MS, Brooks MM, et al. The effect of previous coronary artery bypass surgery on the prognosis of patients with diabetes who have acute myocardial infarction. N Engl J Med 2000;342:989-97.

225. Stone GW, Marsalese D, Brodie BR, et al. A prospective, randomized evaluation of prophylactic intraaortic balloon counterpulsation in high risk patients with acute myocardial infarction treated with primary angioplasty. Second Primary Angioplasty in Myocardial Infarction (PAMI-II) Trial Investigators. J Am Coll Cardiol 1997;29:1459-67.

226. Ohman EM, George BS, White CJ, et al, for the Randomized IABP Study Group. Use of aortic counterpulsation to improve sustained coronary artery patency during acute myocardial infarction: results of a randomized trial. Circulation 1994;90:792-799.

227. Dreifus LS, Fisch C, Griffin JC, et al. Guidelines for implantation of cardiac pacemakers and antiarrhythmia devices: a report of the American College of Cardiology/ American Heart Association task force on assessment of diagnostic and therapeutic cardiovascular procedures (committee on pacemaker implantation). J Am Coll Cardiol 1991;18:1-13.

228. Moss AJ, Hall WJ, Cannom DS, et al, for the Multicenter Automatic Defibrillator Implantation Trial Investigators. Improved survival with an implanted defibrillator in patients with coronary disease at high risk for ventricular arrhythmia. N Engl J Med 1996;335:1933-1940.

229. Buxton AE, Lee KL, Fisher JD, et al, for the Multicenter Unsustained Tachycardia

Trial Investigators. A randomized study of the prevention of sudden death in patients with coronary artery disease. N Engl J Med 1999;341:1882-1890.

230. Moss AJ, Zareba W, Hall WJ, et al. Prophylactic implantation of a defibrillator in patients with myocardial infarction and reduced ejection fraction. N Engl J Med 2002;346:877-83.

231. Freed M, Grines C. In: Essentials of Cardiovascular Medicine, Physicians' Press, Royal Oak, MI, 1994.

232. Jain A, Myers GH, Sapin PM, O'Rourke RA. Comparison of symptom-limited and low level exercise tolerance tests early after myocardial infarction. J Am Coll Cardiol 1993;22:1816-20.

233. Crimm A, Severance HW, Coffey K, et al. Prognostic significance of isolated sinus tachycardia during the first three days of acute myocardial infarction. Am J Med 1984;76:983.

234. Pantridge JF, Adgey AAJ. Pre-hospital coronary care: the mobile coronary care unit. Am J Cardiol 1969;24:666.

235. Graner LE, Gershen BJ, Orlando MM, et al. Bradycardia and its complications in the pre-hospital phase of acute myocardial infarction. Am J Cardiol 1973;32:607.

236. Mark AL. The Bezold-Jarisch reflex revisted: clinical implications of inhibitory reflexes originating in the heart. J Am Coll Cardiol 1983;1:90.

237. Koren G, Weiss AT, Ben-David J, et al. Bradycardia and hypotension following reperfusion with streptokinase (Bezold-Jarish reflex): a sign of coronary thrombolysis and myocardial salvage. Am Heart J 1986;112:468.

238. Berisso MZ, Carratino L, Ferroni A, et al. Frequency, characteristics and significance of supraventricular tachyarrhythmias detected by 24-hour electrocardiographic recording in the late hospital phase of acute myocardial infarction. Am J Cardiol 1990;65:1064.

239. DeSanctis RW, Block P, Hutter AM. Tachyarrhythmias in myocardial infarction. Circulation 1972;45:681.

240. Goldberg RJ, Seeley D, Becker RC, et al. Impact of atrial fibrillation on the in-hospital and long-term survival of patients with acute myocardial infarction: a community-wide perspective. Am Heart J 1990;119:996-1001.

241. Behar S, Zahavi Z, Goldbourt U, Reicher-Reiss H. Long-term prognosis of patients with paroxysmal atrial fibrillation complicating acute myocardial infarction: SPRINT study group. Eur Heart J 1992;13:45-50.

242. Kyriakidis M, Barbetseas J, Antonopoulos A, et al. Early atrial arrhythmias in acute myocardial infarction: role of the sinus node artery. Chest 1992;101:944-947.

243. Serrano CV, Ramires JAF, Mansur AP, et al. Importance of the time of onset of supraventricular tachyarrhythmias on prognosis of patients with acute myocardial infarction. Clin Cardiol 1995;18:84.

244. Crenshaw BS, Ward SR, Stebbins AL, et al. Risk factors and outcomes in patients with atrial fibrillation following acute myocardial infarction. Circulation 1995;92(suppl):I-777.

245. Dhurandhar RW, MacMillan RL, Brown KW. Primary ventricular fibrillation complicating acute myocardial infarction. Am J Cardiol 1971;27:347-351.

246. Lie KI, Wellens HJ, Durrer D. Characteristics and predictability of primary ventricular fibrillation. Eur J Cardiol 1974;1:379-384.

247. Soloman SD, Ridker PM, Antman EM. Ventricular arrhythmias in trials of thrombolytic therapy for acute myocardial infarction: a meta-analysis. Circulation 1993;88:2575-2581.

248. Guidelines 2000 for Cardiopulmonary Resuscitation and Emergency Cardiovascular Care. Circulation 2000;102:I86-I203.

248a. Crenshaw BS, Ward SR, Granger CB, et al. Atrial fibrillation in the setting of acute myocardial infarction: the GUSTO-I experience. Global Utilization of Streptokinase and TPA for Occluded Coronary Arteries. J Am Coll Cardiol 1997;30:406-13.

249. Eldar M, Sievner Z, Goldbourt U, et al. Primary ventricular tachycardia in acute myocardial infarction: clinical characteristics and mortality. The SPRINT study group. Ann Intern Med 1992;117:31.

250. Campbell RWF. Arrhythmias. In: Julian DG, Braunwald E, eds. Management of Acute Myocardial Infarction. London, England: WB Saunders Co Ltd; 1994:223-240.

251. Nordehaug JE, von der Lippe G. Hypokalaemia and ventricular fibrillation in acute myocardial infarction. Br Heart J 1983;50:525-529.

252. Higham PD, Adams PC, Murray A, Campbell RW. Plasma potassium, serum magnesium and ventricular fibrillation: a prospective study. Q J Med 1993;86:609-617.

253. Volpi A, Cavalli A, Santoro E, Tognoni G. Incidence and prognosis of secondary ventricular fibrillation in acute myocardial infarction: evidence for a protective effect of thrombolytic therapy. GISSI Investigators. Circulation 1990;82:1279-1288.

254. Campbell RW, Murray A, Julian DG. Ventricular arrhythmias in trials of thrombolytic therapy for acute myocardial infarction: natural history study. Br Heart J 1981;46:351-357.

255. Antman EM, Berlin JA. Declining incidence of ventricular fibrillation in myocardial infarction: implications for the prophylactic use of lidocaine. Circulation 1992;86:764-773.

256. Behar S, Goldbourt U, Reicher-Reiss H, Kaplinsky E. Prognosis of acute

myocardial infarction complicated by primary ventricular fibrillation: principal investigators of the SPRINT study. Am J Cardiol 1990;66:1208-1211.

257. McMachon S, Collins R, Koster RW, Yusuf S. Effects of prophylactic lidocaine in suspected acute myocardial infarction: an overview of results from the randomized, controlled trials. JAMA 1988;260:1910-1916.

258. Berger PB, Rucco NA Jr, Ryan TJ, et al. Incidence and prognostic implications of heart block complicating inferior myocardial infarction treated with thrombolytic therapy: Results from TIMI II. J Am Coll Cardiol 1992;20:533.

259. McDonald K, O'Sullivan JJ, Conroy RM, et al. Heart block as a predictor of in-hospital death in both acute inferior and acute anterior myocardial infarction. Q J Med 1990;74:277.

260. Clemmensen P, Bates ER, Califf RM, et al. Complete atrioventricular block complicating inferior wall acute myocardial infarction treated with reperfusion therapy: TAMI study group. Am J Cardiol 1991;67:225.

261. Kostuk WJ, Beanlands DS. Complete heart block associated with acute myocardial infarction. Am J Cardiol 1970;26:380.

262. Hindman MC, Wagner GS, Jaro M, et al. The clinical significance of bundle branch block complicating acute myocardial infarction. 2. Indications for temporary and permanent pacemaker insertion. Circulation 1978;58:689.

263. Hindman MC, Wagner GS, Jaro M, et al. The clinical significance of bundle branch block complicating acute myocardial infarction. 1. Clinical characteristics, hospital mortality, and one-year follow-up. Circulation 1978;58:679.

264. Scheinman MM, Gonzalez RP. Fascicular block and acute myocardial infarction. JAMA 1980;224:2646.

265. Klein RC, Vera Z, Mason DT. Intraventricular conduction defects in acute myocardial infarction: incidence, prognosis and therapy. Am Heart J 1984;108:1007.

266. Ricou F, Nicod P, Gilpin E, et al. Influence of a right bundle branch block on short- and long-term survival after acute anterior myocardial infarction. J Am Coll Cardiol 1991;17:858.

267. Ricou F, Nicod P, Gilpin E, et al. Influence of a right bundle branch block on short- and long-term survival after inferior Q-wave myocardial infarction. Am J Cardiol 1991;67:1143.

268. Mullins CB, Atkins JM. Prognoses and management of ventricular conduction blocks in acute myocardial infarction. Mod Concepts Cardiovasc Dis 1976;45:129.

269. Brilakis ES, Wright RS, Kobecky SL, et al. Bundle branch block as a predictor of long-term survival after acute myocardial infarction. Am J Cardiol 2001;88:205-9.

270. Abrams DL, Edelist A, Lruia MH, et al. Ventricular aneurysm: a reappraisal based on a study of 65 consecutive autopsied cases. Circulation 1963;27:164.

271. Meizlish JL, Berger HJ, Plankey M, et al. Functional left ventricular aneurysm formation after acute anterior transmural myocardial infarction: incidence, natural history, and prognostic implications. N Engl J Med 1984;311:1001.

272. Visser CA, Kan G, Meltzer RS, et al. Incidence, timing and prognostic value of left ventricular aneurysm formation after myocardial infarction; a prospective, serial echocardiographic study of 158 patients. Am J Cardiol 1985;57:729-32.

273. Brown SL, Gropler RJ, Harris KM. Distinguishing left ventricular aneurysm from pseudoaneurysm. A review of the literature. Chest 1997;111:1403-09.

274. Komeda M, David TE, Malik A, et al. Operative risks and long-term results of operation for left ventricular aneurysm. Ann Thorac Surg 1992;53:22-58.

275. Frances C, Romero A, Grady D. Left ventricular pseudoaneurysm. J Am Coll Cardiol 1998;32:557-61.

276. Prieto A, Eisenberg J, Thakur RK. Nonarrhythmic complications of acute myocardial infarction. Emerg Med Clin North Am 2001;19:397-415, xii-xiii.

277. Packer M. Heart failure. In: Goldman L, and Bennett JC (eds) Cecil Textbook of Medicine. WB Saunders Co, Philadelphia, 2000, pp. 215-225.

278. Cohn JN. Hormones, drugs, remodeling and outcome in heart failure and after myocardial infarction. Cardiovasc Drugs Ther 2001;15:9-10.

279. Keeley EC, Hillis LD. Left ventricular mural thrombus after acute myocardial infarction. Clin Cardiol 1996;19:83.

280. Halperin JL, Fuster V. Left ventricular thrombi and cerebral embolism. N Engl J Med 1989;320:392.

281. Halperin JL, Peterson P. Thrombosis in the cardiac chambers: ventricular dysfunction and atrial fibrillation. In: Fuster V, and Verstraete M (eds). Thrombosis in Cardiovascular Disorders. Philadelphia, WB Saunders Company, 1992, p.215.

282. Clements SD Jr, Story WE, Hurst JW, et al. Ruptured papillary muscle, a complication of myocardial infarction: clinical presentation, diagnosis and treatment. Clin Cardiol 1985;8:93-103.

283. Tepe NA, Edmunds LH Jr. Operation for acute postinfarction mitral insufficiency and cardiogenic shock. J Thorac Cardiovasc Surg 1985;89:525-530.

284. Kishon Y, Oh JK, Schaff HV, et al. Mitral valve operation in post-infarction rupture of a papillary muscle: immediate results and long-term follow-up of 22 patients. Mayo Clin Proc 1992;67:1023-1030.

285. Piertro A, Eisenberg J, Thakur RK. Nonarrhythmic complications of acute myocardial infarction. Emerg Med Clin North Am 2001;19:397-415, xii-xiii.

285a. Tcheng JE, Jackman JD Jr, Nelson CL, et al. Outcome of patients sustaining acute ischemic mitral regurgitation during myocardial infarction. Ann Intern Med 1992;117:18-24.

285b. Rankin JS, Livesey SA, Smith LR, et al. Trends in the surgical treatment of ischemic mitral regurgitation: effects of mitral valve repair on hospital mortality. Semin Thorac & Cardiovasc Surg 1989;1:149-63.

286. Berman J, Haffajee CI, Alpert JS. Therapy of symptomatic pericarditis after myocardial infarction: retrospective and prospective studies of aspirin, indomethacin, prednisone, and spontaneous resolution. Am Heart J 1981;101:750-753.

287. Lilavie CJ, Gersh PJ. Mechanical and electrical complications of acute myocardial infarction. Mayo Clin Proc 1990;65:709-730.

288. Friedman PL, Brown EJ Jr, Gunther S, et al. Coronary vasoconstrictor effect of indomethacin in patients with coronary-artery disease. N Engl J Med. 1981;305:1171-1175.

289. Hammerman H, Schoen FJ, Braunwald E, Kloner RA. Drug-induced expansion of infarct: morphologic and functional correlations. Circulation 1984;69:611-617.

290. Bulkey BH, Roberts WC. Steroid therapy during acute myocardial infarction: a cause of delayed healing and of ventricular aneurysm. Am J Med 1974;56:244-250.

291. Kloner RA, Fishbein MC, Lew H, Maroko PR, Braunwald E. Mummification of the infarcted myocardium by high dose of corticosteroids. Circulation 1978;57:56-73.

292. Brown EJ Jr, Kloner RA, Schoen FJ, et al. Scar thinning due to ibuprofen administration after experimental myocardial infarction. Am J Cardiol

1983;51:877.

293. Silverman HW, and Pfeifer ME. Relation between use of anti-inflammatory agents and left ventricular free wall rupture during acute myocardial infarction. Am J Cardiol 1987;59:363.

294. Dressler W. The post-myocardial infarction syndrome: a report of forty-four cases. Arch Intern Med 1959;103:28.

295. Lichstein E, Arsura E, Hollander G, et al. Current incidence of postmyocardial infarction (Dressler's) syndrome. Am J Cardiol 1982;50:1269.

296. Khan AH. The postcardiac injury syndromes. Clin Cardiol 1992;15:67.

297. Weisman HF, Healy B. Myocardial infarct expansion, infarct extension, and reinfarction: pathophysiologic concepts. Prog Cardiovasc Dis 1987;30:73-110.

298. The GUSTO investigators. An international randomized trial comparing four thrombolytic strategies for acute myocardial infarction. N Engl J Med 1993;329:673-682.

299. Hutchins GM, Bulkley BH. Infarct expansion versus extension: two different complications of acute myocardial infarction. Am J Cardiol 1978;41:1127-1132.

300. Yusuf S, Wittes J, Friedman L. Overview of results of randomized clinical trials in heart disease: I. Treatments following myocardial infarction. JAMA 1988;260:2088-2093.

301. Zehender M, Kasper W, Kauder E, et al. Right ventricular infarction as an independent predictor of prognosis after acute inferior myocardial infarction. N Engl J Med 1993;328:981-988.

302. Anderson HR, Falk E, Nielsen D. Right ventricular infarction: frequency, size and topography in coronary heart disease: a prospective study comprising 107 consecutive autopsies from a coronary care unit. J Am Coll Cardiol 1987;10:1223-1232.

303. Robalino BD, Whitlow PL, Underwood DA, Salcedo EE. Electrocardiographic manifestations of right ventricular infarction. Am Heart J 1989;118:138-144.

304. Dell'Italia LJ, Starling MR, Blumhardt R, et al. Comparative effects of volume loading, dobutamine, and nitroprusside in patients with predominant right ventricular infarction. Circulation 1985;72:1327-1335.

305. Berger PB, Ruocco NA Jr, Ryan TJ, et al. Frequency and significance of right ventricular dysfunction during inferior wall left ventricular myocardial infarction treated with thrombolytic therapy (results from the Thrombolysis in Myocardial Infarction [TIMI] II trial): the TIMI research group. Am J Cardiol 1993;71:1148-1152.

306. Fijewski TR, Pollack ML, Chan TC, Brady WJ. Electrocardiographic manifestations: right ventricular infarction. J Emerg Med 2002;22:189-94.

307. Lupi-Herrera E, Lasses LA, Cosio-Aranda J, et al. Acute right ventricular infarction: clinical spectrum, results of reperfusion therapy and short-term prognosis. Coron Artery Dis 2002;13:57-64.

308. Fijewski TR, Pollack ML, Chan TC, Brady WJ. Electrocardiographic manifestations: right ventricular infarction. J Emerg Med 2002;22:189-94.

309. Lim ST, Goldstein JA. Right Ventricular Infarction. Current treatment options in cardiovascular medicine. 2001;3:95-101.

310. Mehta SR, Eikelboom JW, Natarajan MK, et al. Impact of right ventricular involvement on mortality and morbidity in patients with inferior myocardial infarction. J Am Coll Cardiol 2001;37:37-43.

311. Haji SA, Movahed A. Right ventricular infarction--diagnosis and treatment. Clin Cardiol 2000;23:473-82.

312. Prieto A, Eisenberg J, Thakur RK. Nonarrhythmic complications of acute

myocardial infarction. Emerg Med Clin North Am 2001 May;19(2):397-415, xii-xiii.

313. Yusuf S, Wittes J, Friedman L. Overview of results of randomized clinical trials in heart disease: I. Treatments following myocardial infarction. JAMA 1988;260:2088-2093.

314. Pollak H, Nobis H, Mlczoch J. Frequency of left ventricular free wall rupture complicating acute myocardial infarction since the advent of thrombolysis. Am J Cardiol 1994;74:184-186.

315. Balakumaran K, Verbaan CJ, Essed CE, et al. Ventricular free wall rupture: sudden, subacute, slow, sealed and stabilized varieties. Eur Heart J 1984;5:282-288.

316. Reardon MJ, Carr CL, Diamond A, et al. Ischemic left ventricular free wall rupture: prediction, diagnosis and treatment. Ann Thoracic Surg 1997;64:1509-13.

317. Califf RM, Bengtson JR. Cardiogenic shock. N Engl J Med 1994;330:1724-30.

318. Hollenberg SM, Kavinsky CJ, Parrillo JE. Cardiogenic shock. Ann Intern Med 1999;131:47-59.

319. Lemery R, Smith HC, Guiliani ER, Gersh BJ. Prognosis in rupture of the ventricular septum after acute myocardial infarction and the role of early surgical intervention. Am J Cardiol 1992;70:147-151.

320. Skillington PD, Davies RH, Luff AJ, et al. Surgical treatment for infarct-related ventricular septal defects: improved early results combined with analysis of late functional status. J Thorac Cardiovasc Surg 1990;99:798-808.

321. Topaz O, Taylor AL. Interventricular septal rupture complicating acute myocardial infarction: from pathophysiologic features to the role of invasive and noninvasive diagnostic modalities in current management. Am J Med 1992;93:683-8.

322. Blanche C, Khan SS, Matloff JM, et al. Results of early repair of ventricular septal defect after an acute myocardial infarction. J Thorac Cardiovasc Surg 1992;104:961-5.

323. Crenshaw BS, Granger CB, Bir Baum Y, et al. Risk factors, angiographic patterns, and outcomes in patients with ventricular septal defect complicating acute myocardial infarction. Circulation 2000;101:27-32.

324. Blanche C, Khan SS, Chaux A, Matloff JM. Postinfarction ventricular septal defect in the elderly: analysis and results. Ann Thorac Surg 1994;57:91-8.

325. Carney RM, Freedland KE, Sheline YI, et al. Depression and coronary heart disease: a review for cardiologists. Clin Cardiol 1997;20:196-200.

325a. Glassman AH, O'Connor CM, Califf RM, et al, for the Sertraline Antidepressant Heart Attack Randomized Trial (SADHART) Group. Sertraline treatment of major depression in patients with acute MI or unstable angina. JAMA 2002;288:701-709.

326. Canto JG, Shlipak MG, Rogers WJ, et al. Prevalence, clinical characteristics, and mortality among patients with myocardial infarction presenting without chest pain. JAMA 2000;283:3223-9.

327. Muller DW, Topol EJ. Selection of patients with acute myocardial infarction for thrombolytic therapy. Ann Intern Med 1990;113:949-60.

328. Granger CB, Hirsch J, Califf RM, et al. Activated partial thromboplastin time and outcome after thrombolytic therapy for acute myocardial infarction: results from the GUSTO-I trial. Circulation 1996;93:870-8.

329. Armstrong PW, Fu Y, Chang WC, et al. Acute coronary syndromes in the GUSTO-IIb trial: prognostic insights and impact of recurrent ischemia. The GUSTO-IIb Investigators. Circulation 1998;98:1860-8.

330. Beta Blocker Heart Attack Study Group. The beta-blocker heart attack trial. JAMA 1981;246:2073-2074.

331. Hjalmarson A, Elmfeldt D, Herlitz J, et al. Effect on mortality of metoprolol in acute myocardial infarction: a double-blind randomized trial. Lancet 1981;2:823-827.

332. Timolol-induced reduction in mortality and reinfarction in patients surviving acute myocardial infarction. N Engl J Med 1981;304:801-807.

333. Gottlieb SS, McCarter RJ, Vogel RA. Effect of beta-blockade on mortality among high-risk and low-risk patients after myocardial infarction. N Engl J Med 1998;339:489-97.

334. Yusuf S, Collins R, MacMahon S, Peto R. Effect of intravenous nitrates on mortality in acute myocardial infarction: an overview of the randomized trials. Lancet 1988;1:1088-92.

335. ISIS-4 (Fourth International Study of Infarct Survival) Collaborative Group. ISIS-4: a randomized factorial trial assessing early oral captopril, oral mononitrate, and intravenous magnesium sulphate in 58,050 patients with suspected acute myocardial infarction. Lancet 1995;345:669-85.

336. GISSI-3: Gruppo Italiano per lo Studio della Sopravvivenza nell'infarto Miocardico. Effects of lisinopril and transdermal glyceryl trinitrate singly and together on 6-week mortality and ventricular function after acute myocardial infarction. Lancet 1994;343:1115-22.

337. ISIS-2 (Second International Study of Infarct Survival) Collaborative Group. Randomized trial of intravenous streptokinase, oral aspirin, both, or neither among 17,187 cases of suspected acute myocardial infarction: ISIS-2. Lancet 1988;2:349-360.

338. Saketkhou BB, Conte FJ, Noris M, et al. Emergency department use of aspirin in patients with possible acute myocardial infarction. Ann Intern Med 1997;127:126-9.

339. Latini R, Maggioni AP, Flather M, et al. ACE-inhibitor use in patients with myocardial infarction: summary of evidence from clinical trials. Circulation 1995;92:3123-3137.

340. Flather MD, Yusuf S, Kober L, et al. Long-term ACE-inhibitor therapy in patients with heart failure or left-ventricular dysfunction: a systematic overview of data from individual patients. Lancet 2000;355:1575-81.

341. Sigurdsson A, Swedberg K. Left ventricular remodeling, neurohormonal activation and early treatment with enalapril (CONSENSUS II) following myocardial infarction. Eur Heart J 1994;15(suppl B):14-19.

342. Cairns JA, Connolly SJ, Roberts R, et al. Randomized trial of outcome after myocardial infarction in patients with frequent or repetitive ventricular premature depolarizations. Lancet 1997;349:675-682.

343. Julian DG, Camm AJ, Frangin G, et al. Randomized trial of effect of amiodarone on mortality in patients with left ventricular dysfunction after recent myocardial infarction. Lancet 1997;349:667-674.

344. Fourth American College of Chest Physicians Consensus Conference on Antithrombotic Therapy. Chest. 1995;108(suppl):225S-522S.

345. Roux S, Christeller S, Ludin E. Effects of aspirin on coronary reocclusion and recurrent ischemia after thrombolysis: a meta-analysis. J Am Coll Cardiol 1992;19:671-7.

346. ISIS-2. ISIS-2 (Second Internation Study of Infarct Survival) Collaborative Group. Randomized trial of intravenous streptokinase, oral aspirin, both, or neither among 17,187 cases of suspected acute myocardial infarction. Lancet

1988;2:349-60.

347. Song KH, Fedyk R, Hoover R. Interaction of ACE inhibitors and aspirin in patients with congestive heart failure. Ann Pharmacother 1999;33:375-7.

348. Latini R, Tognoni G, Maggioni A, et al., for the Angiotensin-converting Enzyme Inhibitor Myocardial Infarction Collaborative Group. Clinical effects of early angiotensin-converting enzyme inhibitor treatment for acute myocardial infarction are similar in the presence and absence of aspirin. Systematic overview of individual data from 96,712 randomized patients. J Am Coll Cardiol 2000;35:1801-1807.

349. Catella-Lawson F, Reilly MP, Kapoor SC, et al. Cyclooxygenase inhibitors and the antiplatelet effects of aspirin. N Engl J Med 2001;345:1809-17.

350. Yusuf S, Peto R, Lewis J, et al. Beta blockade during and after myocardial infarction: an overview of the randomized trials. Prog Cardiovasc Dis 1985;27:335-371.

351. Norris RM, Barnaby PF, Brown MA, et al. Prevention of ventricular fibrillation during acute myocardial infarction by intravenous propranolol. Lancet 1984;2:883-6.

352. Roberts R, Rogers WJ, Mueller HS, et al. Immediate versus deferred beta-blockade following thrombolytic therapy in patients with acute myocardial infarction. Results of the Thrombolysis in Myocardial Infarction (TIMI) II-B study. Circulation 1991;83:422-37.

353. First International Study of Infarct Survival Collaborative Group. Randomized trial of intravenous atenolol among 16,027 cases of suspected acute myocardial infarction. ISIS-1. Lancet 1986;2:57-66.

354. Yusuf S, Wittes J, Friedman L. Overview of results of randomized clinical trials in heart disease, II: unstable angina, heart failure, primary prevention with aspirin, and risk factor modification. JAMA 1988;260:2259-63.

355. Yusuf S, Peto R, Lewis J, et al. Beta blockade during and after myocardial infarction: an overview of the randomized trials. Prog Cardiovasc Dis 1985;27:335-71.

356. Muller JE, Morrison J, Stone PH, et al. Nifedipine therapy for patients with threatened and acute myocardial infarction: a randomized, double-blind placebo-controlled comparison. Circulation 1984;69:740-747.

357. Goldbourt U, Behar S, Reicher-Reiss H, et al. Early administration of nifedipine in suspected acute myocardial infarction: the Secondary Prevention Reinfarction Israel Nifedipine Trial 2 Study. Arch Intern Med 1993;153:345-353.

358. Opie LH, Messerli FH. Nifedipine and mortality: grave defects in the dossier. Circulation 1995;92:1068-1073.

359. The Multicenter Diltiazem Postinfarction Trial Research Group. The effect of diltiazem on mortality and reinfarction after myocardial infarction. N Engl J Med 1988;319:385-392.

360. Gibson RS, Boden WE, Theroux P, et al. Diltiazem and reinfarction in patients with non-Q-wave myocardial infarction: results of a double-blind randomized, multicenter trial. N Engl J Med 1986;315:423-429.

361. Boden WE, van Gilst WH, Scheldewaert RG, et al, for the Incomplete Infarction Trial of European Research Collaborators Evaluating Prognosis post-Thrombolysis (INTERCEPT) group. Diltiazem in acute myocardial infarction treated with thrombolytic agents: a randomized placebo-controlled trial. Lancet 2000;355:1751-1756.

362. Hansen JF, Hagerup L, Sigurd B, et al., for the Danish Verapamil Infarction Trial (DAVIT) Study Group. Cardiac event rates after acute myocardial infarction in patients treated with verapamil and trandolapril versus trandolapril alone.

Am J Cardiol 1997;79:738-41.

363. Malmberg K, Ryden L, Efendic S, et al. Randomized trial of insulin-glucose infusion followed by subcutaneous insulin treatment in diabetic patients with acute myocardial infarction (DIGAMI study): effects on mortality at 1 year. J Am Coll Cardiol 1995;26:57-65.

364. Fath-Ordoubadi F, Beatt KJ. Glucose-insulin-potassium therapy for treatment of acute myocardial infarction: an overview of randomized placebo-controlled trials. Circulation 1997;96:1152-1156.

364a. Zijlistra F. Glucose-insulin-potassium study (GIPS). Presented at the European Society of Cardiolgy meeting, Berlin, Germany, Sept. 2002.

365. Eikelboom JW, Anand SS, Malmberg K, et al. Unfractionated heparin and low-molecular-weight heparin in acute coronary syndrome without ST elevation: a meta-analysis. Lancet 2000;355:1936-42.

366. The RISC Group. Risk of myocardial infarction and death during treatment with low dose aspirin and intravenous heparin in men with unstable coronary artery disease. Lancet 1990;336:827-830.

367. Theroux P, Ouirnet H, McCans J, et al. Aspirin, heparin, or both to treat acute unstable angina. N Engl J Med 1988;319:1105-1111.

368. Theroux P, Waters D, Lam J, et al. Reactivation of unstable angina after the discontinuation of heparin. N Engl J Med 1992;327:141-145.

369. Neri Serneri GG, Gensini GF, Poggesi L, et al. Effect of heparin, aspirin, or alteplase in reduction of myocardial ischemia in refractory unstable angina. Lancet 1990;335:615-618.

370. MacMahon S, Collins R, Knight C, et al. Reduction in major morbidity and mortality by heparin in acute myocardial infarction. Circulation. 1988;78(suppl II):II-98.

371. The GUSTO Angiographic Investigators.

The effects of tissue plasminogen activator, streptokinase or both on coronary-artery patency, ventricular function, and survival after acute myocardial infarction. N Engl J Med 1993;329:1615-1622.

372. The International Study Group. In-hospital mortality and clinical course of 20,891 patients with suspected acute myocardial infarction randomized between alteplase and streptokinase with or without heparin. Lancet 1990;336:71-75.

373. The GUSTO Angiographic Investigators. The effects of tissue plasminogen activator, streptokinase or both on coronary-artery patency, ventricular function, and survival after acute myocardial infarction. N Engl J Med 1993;329:1615-1622.

374. Neri Sernen GG, Roveli F, Gensini GF, et al. Effectiveness of low-dose heparin in prevention of myocardial reinfarction. Lancet 1987;1:937-942.

375. The SCATI (Studio sulla Calciparina nell'Angina e nella Thrombosi Ventricolare nell'Infarto) Group. Randomized controlled trial of subcutaneous calcium-heparin in acute myocardial infarction. Lancet 1989;2:182-186.

376. Brieger DB, Mak KH, Kottke-Marchant K, Topol EJ. Heparin induced thrombocytopenia. J Am Coll Cardiol 1998;31:1449-1459.

377. Greinacher A, Lubenow N. Recombinant hirudin in clinical practice. Circulation 2001;103:1479-1484.

378. Teo KK, Yusuf S, Furberg CD. Effects of prophylactic antiarrhythmic drug therapy in acute myocardial infarction: an overview of results from randomized controlled trials. JAMA 1993;270:1589-1595.

379. Teo KK, Yusuf S, Collins R, et al. Effects of intravenous magnesium in suspected acute myocardial infarction:

overview of randomized trials. BMJ 1991;303:1499-1503.

380. Antman EM, Lau J, Kupelnick B, et al. A comparison of results of meta-analysis of randomized control trials and recommendations of clinical experts: treatments for myocardial infarction. JAMA 1992;268:240-248.

381. Woods KL, Fletcher S, Roffe C, Haider Y. Intravenous magnesium sulphate in suspected acute myocardial infarction: results of the second Leicester Intravenous Magnesium Intervention Trial (LIMIT-2). Lancet 1992;339:1553-1558.

382. Woods KL, Fletcher S. Long-term outcome after intravenous magnesium sulphate in suspected acute myocardial infarction: the second Leicester Intravenous Magnesium Intervention Trial (LIMIT-2). Lancet 1994;343:816-819.

383. Shechter M, Hod H, Chouraqui P, et al. Magnesium therapy in acute myocardial infarction when patients are not candidates for thrombolytic therapy. Am J Cardiol 1995;75:321-323.

384. Antman EM. Magnesium in acute MI: timing is critical. Circulation 1995;92:2367-2372.

384a. Antman E. Magnesium in coronaries (MAGIC) trial. Presented at the European Society of Cardiolgy meeting, Berlin, Germany, Sept. 2002.

385. Arsenian MA. Magnesium and cardiovascular disease. Prog Cardiovasc Dis 1993;35:271-310.

386. Woods KL. Possible pharmacological actions of magnesium in acute myocardial infarction. Br J Clin Pharmacol 1991;32:3-10.

387. Yusuf S, Collins R, MacMahon S, Peto R. Effect of intravenous nitrates on mortality in acute myocardial infarction: an overview of the randomized trials. Lancet 1988;1:1088-92.

388. ASPECT Research Group. Effect of long-term oral anticoagulant treatment on mortality and cardiovascular morbidity after myocardial infarction: Anticoagulants in the Secondary Prevention of Events in Coronary Thrombosis (ASPECT) research group. Lancet 1994;343:499-503.

389. A controlled comparison of aspirin and oral anticoagulants in prevention of death after myocardial infarction. N Engl J Med 1982;307:701-8.

390. Meijer A, Verheugt FW, Werter CJ, et al. Aspirin versus coumadin in the prevention of reocclusion and recurrent ischemia after successful thrombolysis: a prospective placebo-controlled angiographic study. Results of the APRICOT study. Circulation 1993;87:1524-30.

391. Organization to Assess Strategies for Ischemic Syndromes (OASIS-2) Investigators. Effects of recombinant hirudin (lepirudin) compared with heparin on death, myocardial infarction, refractory angina, and revascularization procedures in patients with acute myocardial ischemia without ST elevation: a randomized trial. Lancet 1999;353:429-38.

392. Coumadin Aspirin Reinfarction Study (CARS) Investigators. Randomized double-blind trial of fixed low-dose warfarin with aspirin after myocardial infarction. Lancet 1997;350:389-96.

393. Fiore LD, Ezekowitz MD, Brophy MT, et al. Department of Veterans Affairs Cooperative Studies Program Clinical Trial comparing combined warfarin and aspirin with aspirin alone in survivors of acute myocardial infarction. Circulation 2002;105:557-63.

394. van Es RF, Jonker JC, Verheugt FWA, et al. Aspirin and coumadin after acute coronary syndromes (the ASPECT-2 study): a randomised controlled trial. Lancet 2002;360:109-113.

395. Results of the second Warfarin-Aspirin Re-Infarction Study (WARIS II). Presented at the XXIII Congress of the

European Society of Cardiology, Stockholm, Sweden, September, 2001.

396. Brouwer MA, van den Bergh PJPC, Aengevaeren WRM, et al. Aspirin plus coumarin versus aspirin alone in the prevention of reocclusion after fibrinolysis for acute myocardial infarction. Results of the antithrombotics in the prevention of reocclusion in coronary thrombolysis (APRICOT)-2 trial. Circulation [doi:10.1161/01. CIR.0000024408.81821.32]. 2002. Available at: www.circulationaha.org.

397. Ansell JE. Anticoagulation management as a risk factor for adverse events: grounds for improvement. J Thromb Thrombolys 1998;5(suppl):S13-S18.

398. Steinhubl SR, Berger PB, Mann JT III, et al. Early and sustained dual oral antiplatelet therapy following percutaneous coronary intervention. The CREDO trial. JAMA 2002;288:2411-20.

INDEX

Abciximab, see GP IIb/IIIa inhibitors
Accelerated idioventricular rhythm 116
ACE inhibitors 31,148
Acute coronary syndrome, see non-ST-elevation
    ACS, ST-elevation ACS
Adenosine 148
Amiodarone 149-150
Aneurysm, left ventricular 125
Angioplasty, see percutaneous coronary
    intervention (PCI)
Argatroban 92
Aspirin 31,75,150
Atrial fibrillation 113
Atrial flutter 112
Atropine 150-151
AV block
    first degree 117
    second degree
        Type I 118
        Type II 119
    third degree 50,120

Balloon angioplasty, see percutaneous
    coronary intervention (PCI)
Beta-blockers
    acute 30-31,151
    chronic 152
Bundle branch block
    left 13,123
    right 122
    bilateral 124

Calcium antagonists 32,152-153
Cardiac catheterization for risk stratification 105
Cardiac markers 15-17
    non-ST-elevation ACS 61
    ST-elevation ACS 15-17
Cardiac troponins 15-17
Cardiogenic shock 38,135
Clopidogrel 76-79,153-154
    coronary stenting 78
    non-ST-elevation ACS 76-77
    secondary prevention 79
Coronary artery bypass grafting . 38-39,74,99
Creatine kinase 15

Depression 137
Direct thrombin inhibitors 91-92
Dobutamine 154

Dopamine 154-155
Dressler's syndrome 132

Echocardiogram for risk stratification 104
Electrocardiogram
    non-ST-elevation ACS 6,59
    ST-elevation ACS 4,13-15
Electrophysiology study for risk stratification 104
Enoxaparin, see low-molecular-weight
    heparin
Epinephrine 155
Eptifibatide, see GP IIb/IIIa inhibitors

Failed fibrinolysis 125
Fibrinolytic therapy 40-55,155
    adjunctive antithrombin therapy 48
    choice of agents 44
    complications 48-51
    contraindications 43
    goal of therapy 40
    indications 43
    limitations 42
    new strategies 53-55
    rPA 44-45
    streptokinase 44-45
    time-dependent benefits 42
    TNK-tPA 44, 46
    tPA 44-45
Furosemide 156

Glucose-insulin-potassium 156
GP IIb/IIIa inhibitors . . 33-36,73-74,79-85,156
    adjunct to fibrinolysis 53
    adjunct to PCI
        non-ST-elevation ACS 73-74
        ST-elevation ACS 33,35-36
    bleeding 81
    dosing 83
    emergency CABG 84-85
    mechanism of action 79-80
    non-ST-elevation ACS 79-85
    thrombocytopenia 84
    trials 82
    types of inhibitors 79-81,83

Heart failure, acute 126
Heparin
    low-molecular-weight see low-molecular-
        weight heparin

unfractionated 158-159
  adjunct to fibrinolysis 45-46,48-49
  adjunct to GP IIb/IIIa inhibitors 84
  adjunct to PCI 37-38
Holter monitor for risk stratification 104

Ibutilide 159
Immediate PCI (patent vessel) 98
Implantable cardioverter-defibrillator 101
Intra-aortic balloon pump 99
Intra-arterial pressure monitoring 103
Isolated hemiblock 121

Left ventricular
  aneurysm 125
  dysfunction 126
  pseudoaneurysm 126
  thrombus 127
Lepirudin 92
Lidocaine 158
Low-molecular-weight heparin
  non-ST-elevation ACS 85-91,157
    complications 89
    dose 89
    indications 89
    mechanism of action 85,88
    recommendations 90
    trials 86,90-91
    vs. unfractionated heparin 86-87
  ST-elevation ACS
    adjunct to fibrinolytic therapy 48
    adjunct to PCI 37

Magnesium sulfate 160
Major depression 137
Mitral regurgitation
  ischemic papillary muscle 130
  ruptured papillary muscle 130
Morphine sulfate 160
Myocardial infarction, see non-ST-elevation
  ACS, ST-elevation ACS
  right ventricular 133
Myoglobin 15-17

Nitroglycerin
  acute 160-161
  chronic 161-162
Nitroprusside 162
Non-ST-elevation ACS 58-95
  cardiac markers 61
  diagnosis 58
  electrocardiogram 59-60
  general measures 63-70

  emergency department 63-67
  hospital management 67-69
  post-discharge 69-70
  interventional management
    CABG 74
    early invasive vs. early conservative 70-73
    GP IIb/IIIa inhibitors 73-74
    stents vs. PTCA 73
  medical therapy
    aspirin 75
    clopidogrel 76-79
    direct thrombin inhibitors 91-92
    GP IIb/IIIa inhibitors 79-85
    low-molecular-weight heparin ... 85-91
    statins 92-93
  overview 63
  risk stratification 61-62
  symptoms 59

Oxygen 162

Pacemaker 32,100
  permanent 100
  temporary 100
Papillary muscle
  ischemic 130
  ruptured 130
Percutaneous coronary intervention (PCI)
  non-ST-elevation ACS 70-74
    early invasive vs. early conservative
      approaches 67-68,70-73
    GP IIb/IIIa inhibitors 73-74
    PTCA vs. stents 73
  ST-elevation ACS 33-39
    adjunctive pharmacotherapy 36-37
    cardiogenic shock 38
    deficiencies 37
    direct 97
    post-lytic therapy 51-53
      delayed 52
      immediate 51
      recurrent ischemia 53
      rescue 51
    PTCA vs. fibrinolysis 26
    PTCA vs. stents 27,33-34
    technique, procedural 37
Pericarditis 131-132
  acute 131
  Dressler's syndrome 132
Posterior MI 14
Primary PCI 97
Prinzmetal's angina 95
Procainamide 162-163

Pseudoaneurysm 126
PTCA, see percutaneous coronary
   intervention (PCI)
Pulmonary artery catheterization 101-102

Recurrent Ischemia 53,132
Reinfarction 132
Rescue PCI 51, 98
Right ventricular infarction 133
rPA 44-45
Rupture, cardiac 134

Shock, cardiogenic 38,135
Signal-averaged ECG 104
Sinus bradycardia 50,110
Sinus pause/arrest 111
Sinus tachycardia 109
ST-elevation ACS 12-56
  cardiac markers 15-17
  complications, see individual complications
  diagnosis . . . .
    electrocardiogram 13-15
  fibrinolytic therapy 18-26, 40-56
  general measures 29-32
    early hospitalization 30
    emergency department 29
    late hospitalization 30
    post-discharge 30
  interventional management, see PCI for
    ST-elevation ACS
  monitoring 102-103
  non-medical therapy 97-103
  percutaneous coronary intervention 26
    deficiencies 37
    intraprocedural drug therapy 36-37
    preprocedural drug therapy 36
    technique 37
  PTCA vs. fibrinolysis 26
  PTCA vs. stents 27,33-34
  risk stratification 103-107
  symptoms 12
Statins 92-93,163
Stents, see percutaneous coronary intervention
  drug-eluting 35
Streptokinase 44-45
Symptoms
  non-ST-elevation ACS 59
  ST-elevation ACS 12

Thrombolytic therapy, see fibrinolytic therapy
Thrombus, left ventricular 127
Tirofiban, see GP IIb/IIIa inhibitors
TNK-tPA 44, 46

tPA 44-45
Trials
  ACUTE-2 86
  ADMIRAL 35
  APRICOT-2 162
  ASPECT-2 162
  ASSENT-2 44
  ASSENT-3 53-55
  BARI 99
  CADILLAC 34, 35
  CAMIAT 149
  CAPRIE 77
  CAPTURE 82
  CARS 162
  CHAMP 93
  CLASSICS 77
  CONSENSUS-2 155
  CPORT 28
  CRUISE 86
  CURE 76-77
  DANAMI-2 41
  DAVIT 152
  DIGAMI 155
  ELUTES 35
  EMIAT 149
  EPIC 82
  EPILOG 82
  EPISTENT 82
  ESPRIT 82
  ESSENCE 90
  FRAXIS 91
  FRESCO 34
  FRIC 91
  FRISC-2 70-71
  GIPS 155
  GISSI-1 18
  GISSI-3 160
  GUSTO I 40,44
  GUSTO III 44
  GUSTO IV ACS 82
  GUSTO V 54,56
  HERO-2 48
  HOPE 148
  IMPACT-2 82
  IMPACT-AMI 53
  INTERACT 85,156
  ISAR 35
  ISIS-4 160
  MADIT 101
  MADIT-2 101
  MAGIC 159
  MDPIT 152
  MIRACL 92

MUSTT 101
NICE-1, 3, 4 86
OASIS-2 162
OAT 52
PACT 36,51

Trials *(continued)*
PARADIGM 53
PARAGON 82
PASTA 34
PCI-CURE 77
PRAGUE 41
PRAGUE-2 41
PRISM-PLUS 73
PURSUIT 73
RAPPORT 82
RAVEL 35
RESTORE 82
RITA-3 71
SHOCK 38
SIRIUS 35
SPEED 53
STENT-PAMI 33-34

STOPAMI 34
SWIFT 52
SYNERGY 65,85,90
TACTICS-TIMI 18 71
TAMI-6 52
TAMI-8 53
TARGET 67
TIMI 2B 52
TIMI 3B 70,72
TIMI 11B 90
TIMI 14a pilot 53
WARIS-2 162
VANQWISH 70-71
Troponins, cardiac 15-17

Unstable angina, *see non-ST-elevation ACS*

Ventricular fibrillation 115
Ventricular septal defect 136
Ventricular tachycardia 51,114

Warfarin 163-164

ACS ESSENTIALS — ORDERING INFORMATION

Price (U.S. dollars)
1–9 copies: $16.95 each
10–49 copies: $15.95 each
50–100 copies: $14.95 each
> 100 copies: call

Shipping
<u>USA</u>: UPS Ground delivery
1–3 copies: add $5
4–10 copies: add $7
10–49 copies: add $10
50–100 copies: add $15
> 100 copies: call

Call for next day, 2-day, or 3-day express delivery charges

<u>Outside USA</u>: Call, fax, or e-mail for delivery charges

Michigan residents: add 6%

4 Ways to Order:
By Internet: www.physicianspress.com
By Phone: (248) 616-3023
By Fax:*   (248) 616-3003
By Mail:*   Physicians' Press
        620 Cherry Avenue
        Royal Oak, Michigan 48073

*   Please print or type name, mailing address, credit card number and expiration date or purchase order number (if applicable), telephone number (important), fax number, and e-mail address. We accept VISA, MasterCard, and American Express.

Visit our website at www.physicianspress.com

- Hypertension Essentials 2003
- Dyslipidemia Essentials 2003
- Essentials of Cardiovascular Medicine 2003
- Antibiotic Essentials 2003
- The Complete Guide to ECGs
- The ECG Criteria Book
- The Manual of Interventional Cardiology
- Other Titles, Quizzes, Reviews

PHYSICIANS' PRESS

Innovative Medical Publishing